HEALTH TIPS, MYTHS, AND TRICKS

A Physician's Advice

Health information to liberate us from "Snake Oil"

Morton E. Tavel, MD

*To Sandra Leach,
with best personal regards,
Morton Tavel MD*

Brighton Publishing LLC
435 N. Harris Drive
Mesa, AZ 85203

HEALTH TIPS, MYTHS, AND TRICKS

A Physician's Advice

Health information to liberate us from "Snake Oil"

Morton E. Tavel, MD

Brighton Publishing LLC
435 N. Harris Drive
Mesa, AZ 85203
www.BrightonPublishing.com

ISBN13: 978-1-62183-340-6

ISBN 10: 1-62183-340-2

Printed in the United States of America

Copyright © 2015

First Edition

Cover Design: Tom Rodriguez

Reviews

"Whether you read "Health Tips, Myths and Tricks" straight through, or jump around to the topics where you really need someone to blow through the myths and unscientific claims—chocolate and health? Fish during pregnancy? Losing weight? Cranberry juice and UTIs?, you'll come away not only smarter about specific subjects but better able to cut through the BS the next time a crazy health claim comes along. For you know it will."

~Sharon Begley

Senior science writer at STAT, the life sciences publication of the Boston Globe. Previously she was the senior health & science correspondent at Reuters (2012-2015), the science editor and the science columnist at Newsweek (2007 to 2011), and a contributing writer at the magazine and its website, The Daily Beast (2011). From 2002 to 2007, she was the science columnist at The Wall Street Journal, and previous to that the science editor at Newsweek. She is the co-author (with Richard J. Davidson) of the 2012 book The Emotional Life of Your Brain, the author of the 2007 book Train Your Mind, Change Your Brain, and the co-author (with Jeffrey Schwartz) of the 2002 book The Mind and the Brain. She is the recipient of numerous awards for her writing, including an honorary degree from the University of North Carolina at Asheville for communicating science to the public, and the Public Understanding of Science Award from the San Francisco Exploratorium.

"This book should be subtitled "Fact-checking the snake-oil salesmen." Snopes.com and factcheck.org allow us to check the credibility of the dubious "news items" that populate the internet; this book provides a similar service for all of us who are susceptible to claims that we desperately want to believe ("If you just avoid eating this one food, you'll lose weight without dieting.") Dr. Tavel has done the due diligence that most of us don't—or can't—do, and has tested the constant hucksterism with which we are all inundated against sound science. (No, vaccines do not cause autism...). This accessible and useful compendium should join the other reference books in your library."

~Sheila Kennedy

Author and Professor, School of Public and Environmental Affairs, Director, Indiana University Center for Civic Literacy.

"We live in a world with rampant misinformation when it comes to health, fitness, and nutrition. Dr. Tavel does a thorough job of mitigating many of the myths out there in this book by backing up his opinions with solid research."

~Kimberly Dawn Neumann

Writer, Performer, Health and Fitness professional

"Chock full of practical advice that can help people protect their heath and avoid wasting money."

~Stephen Barrett, editor of website, Quackwatch, and consumer advocate, vice-president of the Institute for Science in Medicine and a Fellow of the Committee for Skeptical inquiry.

⧼Table of Contents⧽

Myths

Tricks

ᴄ⌒Introduction⌒ᴐ

T his book consists of three parts:

1. The first section: Tips, is about health and wellness that can be incorporated into one's daily life, that hopefully will create a healthier and longer physical outlook, less waste of money, and maybe even lower body weight (if you are one of those many with excess fat storage).

2. The second section: Myths, are common misconceptions about almost anything regarding our physical makeup and how we relate to the world around us.

3. The third section: Tricks, is devoted to various stratagems that are designed to take your money in exchange for useless—or dangerous—products or information.

Despite division into three sections, there is in fact much overlap, because if one believes many of the myths, this may cause one to forego measures (tips) that may have afforded better health. On the other hand, mythical beliefs may cause us to fall easy prey to those dreaded scams that we all desire to avoid.

After scanning the chapter titles, the reader may wish to concentrate on those of special interest; nevertheless, I have tried to create all chapters to contain some helpful information for as wide an audience as possible. To do so, I have drawn from an eclectic collection of material that includes my personal biomedical background, scientific publications, media reports deemed accurate, and many other trustworthy sources. If some sources have been overlooked, it was unintentional. In all cases I have endeavored to seek the most reliable and scientifically documented information.

My initial motivation for creating this book was derived from my research used in preparation of my previous book entitled "Snake Oil is Alive and Well. The Clash between Myths and Reality. Reflections of a Physician."

In that book, I attempted to provide the reader with not only specific examples of the misleading information being foisted off on the public, but also the tools to recognize the common fallacies in the thought processes that allowed such falsehoods to flourish. After completing that book, I realized there were many subjects that extended beyond merely "snake oil," i.e., the metaphorical expression that encompassed useless remedies of all sorts. In the process, I encountered not only additional widespread myths and scams, but much additional information of positive value for public consumption.

Tips

ᴄᴀChapter 1ᴇᴅ

Aids to Losing Weight: Some Effective, Some Useless, Some Dangerous

With about 70% of the U.S. population either overweight or frankly obese, everyone seems to be seeking ways to shed excess blubber. In the process, they often seek any way to accomplish this without troubling to reduce caloric intake, i.e., dieting. Wouldn't that be great, but what are the actual facts, and who is actually overweight?

In the health professions, we often use the so-called body mass index, (BMI) to determine the presence and amount of overweight, which is simply a way of combining height with weight to yield a single number, or index. The easiest way to find your own index is to view the chart below[1]. Simply find your weight on the horizontal axis, then your height on the vertical axis, and connect the lines (you can select from either the metric or English measurement systems). A BMI of 18-25 is considered normal, 25-30, overweight, and everything over 30, frankly obese. But these numbers are only approximate, for other factors, such as proportion of your weight composed of body fat, play a role. For instance, if one is muscular with little body fat, being slightly "overweight" would not mean obesity and not be a danger to health. The distribution of fat also is important, for accumulation of fat around the waist, rather than legs and hips, raises one's ultimate chances of cardiovascular disease, even though total weight may be within the normal range.

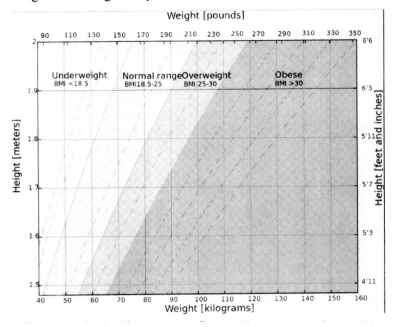

This chart, therefore, gives you at least a rough idea of whether you must lose weight and how many pounds you need to shed to achieve a BMI of 25 or below (without attempting to grow taller).

First we must consider the underlying causes of obesity in our society.

Although this subject is too complex to cover in detail here, a few comments are warranted. We begin by considering the enormous consumption of sugary beverages. So how much does consumption of these drinks contribute to our current obesity? On average, beverages with added sugar constitute over 10% of caloric intake nationwide, and they supply little of nutritional value. That is the first major hurdle and an obvious target for restriction.

Also societal trends require consideration. For instance, studies showing that the ready availability of foods high in sugar, fat, sodium, and calories increase average body weight. Adults living closer to fast food restaurants consume such food more frequently than those who don't and, consequently, are heavier. This is especially important for children; schools that serve more unhealthy foods or provide vending machines with unhealthy foods tend to be heavier than children whose schools do not permit such practices. Similarly, adolescents who attend schools near fast food restaurants are more likely to be obese.

Compounding these problems are other economic forces surrounding foods: The cost per calorie of healthy foods exceeds those of poor nutrient foods. In the past 30 years, this cost disparity has increased; between 1985 and 2000, the prices of healthy foods, like fruits and vegetables, fish, and dairy products increased at more than twice the rate of prices of sugar and sweets, fats and oils, and carbonated beverages.

Finally, we must consider portion sizes as another contributor to obesity. For children alone, between 1977 and 2006 the average portions of soft drinks, pizza, and Mexican foods increased by 34, 140, and 139 calories, respectively. Sodas, sold originally in 6.5 oz. bottles, are now typically sold in 20 ounce containers. Studies have shown in general that increased portion sizes lead to rises in calorie intake: as a result, US adults now consume 500 calories more per day in 2006 than they did in 1977. This trend has been further exacerbated by our increased eating away from home, for in 2008, Americans spent 49% of their food budget on food away from home compared with 33% in 1970. On average, each meal eaten outside the home increases that day's consumption

3

by about 134 calories, while, at the same time shifts the content toward less nutritious ingredients such as saturated fat and added sugar.

Given this sad state of affairs, let's now analyze the four general means used by most people in attempting to shed pounds:

1.   Reduce one's calories through diet (ugh!), a doleful choice, but effective.

2.   Resort to dietary supplements, often touted by slick salesmen, with or without medical qualifications.

3.   Diet pills. There are currently four approved products on the market.

4.   Surgery, the most radical approach for the most massively (morbidly) obese.

The Best Means to Reduce

Reduction of calories by diet clearly emerges as the winner. But how do we best accomplish this? In a comprehensive analysis of 48 diets reported in the American Medical Association journal[2], any diet containing reduced fat or carbohydrate (preferably both) could achieve satisfactory results. From this study the authors concluded; "Significant weight loss was observed with any low-carbohydrate or low-fat diet. Weight loss differences between individual named diets were small. This supports the practice of recommending any diet that a patient will adhere to in order to lose weight." Although the authors did not mention it, the reduction of dietary fat and carbohydrate is usually compensated for by added protein, which, in the process of digestion alone, causes the body to burn about 30% more calories per unit volume than that produced by the other food sources. Thus even though the original calorie content of protein equals that of carbohydrate (and less than half that of fat), the net effect will be the burning up of about 20-30% more caloric energy than equal volumes of carbohydrates and other food sources. Further enhancing its advantages, protein produces a greater—and longer persisting—sense of satiation. That's why time-honored diets such as those of Weight-Watcher's and Jenny Craig tend to achieve success, for, in addition to adding more fruits and vegetables, these diets increase the percentage intake of protein—lean, of course.

But all these dietary modifications must be followed—both in the short and long term, to attain ultimate success. Regular exercise, while usually not causing much weight loss in itself, is an important adjunct to all diets and makes reducing easier. First you must start with a reasonable goal, say reducing by 5% of body weight over a period of one to two months. The first few pounds are usually the most difficult.

Begin by reducing the portion sizes, consuming a total of fewer than 2,000 calories/day. Cook and eat frequently at home, for this provides better control of portion quantities and salt intake.

Increase intake of fruit, vegetables, and protein, for that generally provides satiating bulk with fewer calories per unit of volume. Reduce refined grains in favor of whole grains, and include liberal amounts of lean meats and seafood. As explained in chapter 2, eat breakfast regularly.

Completely eliminate your sugar (sucrose and corn syrup fructose) intake. This means total elimination of all sugary soft drinks in favor of water or unsweetened tea. I discourage the use of artificially sweetened drinks because research has not shown them to be of much help in weight reduction, as explained in chapter 22.

But just plain water provides one potential aid to this approach to weight control. Replacing sweetened drinks with water increases the sensation of fullness and reduces the perception of hunger. Besides being free of calories, water possesses the added advantage of promoting energy expenditure through support of body metabolism. A group from the Berlin School of Public Health[3] reviewed the association between water consumption and weight. They related difference in body weights based upon amount of water consumption. They found that, in individuals attempting to reduce weight through calorie control, increased water consumption reduced body weight after 3-12 months, compared with simple dieting alone. So try preceding each meal with one-half quart (16 oz.) of water. This seems to reduce calorie consumption because of earlier satiety. On average, people who drink this much water before meals eat an average of 75 fewer calories at each meal. That doesn't sound like much, but multiply 75 calories by 365 days a year. Even if you only drink water before dinner every day, you'd consume 27,000 fewer calories over the course of the year. That's almost an eight-pound weight loss.

Obviously, increasing water consumption can only play a secondary contributing role in weight control, for it needs to be combined with other lifestyle and dietary modifications. But at least it's inexpensive, harmless, and, for most people, is worth a try.

Dietary Supplements

Unfortunately, dietary supplements are promoted as products that are safe and effective, but they are rarely either. Since they are not subjected to the rigorous study required of drugs, they are almost universally ineffective, but worse yet, they are often unsafe. Although unable to keep up with the huge number of products, the Food and Drug Administration

(FDA) has recalled hundreds of weight-loss supplements that contained drugs that were usually not listed on labels.

I encounter ads almost daily touting "miracle" supplements claiming to provide weight reduction without dieting. The list goes on and on, but several notable examples are the following: Saffron extract, Garcinia Cambogia, green coffee bean extract, Hydroxycut, OxyElite Pro, MS2 Meltdown, OxyTherm Pro, Sensa, L'Occitane, HCT Diet Direct, acai berry, and yohimbe extract. None of these products has been adequately studied and any or all might be harmful. Side effects may be numerous and dangerous, perhaps most notably liver failure (requiring liver transplantation in some cases and one death of a 19 year-old-man), rhabdomyolysis (extensive muscle breakdown), and kidney failure. Very often these products contain the word "natural" or "herbal," which suggests that they were safer than prescription medication, but nothing could be further from the truth!

Conclusion:

Don't take any weight-loss supplements. They are unregulated, ineffective, but most importantly—they could harm you. Further information about this subject is noted in chapter 55.

Prescription Diet Pills

Before 2010 three weight-loss drugs (Fen-Phen, Acomplia, and Meridia) either had failed to gain FDA approval or were taken off the market because of serious side effects.

At present the following four drugs have been approved, but all with reservations:

The first is Orlistat, provided in both prescription and over-the-counter forms, Xenical^R and Alli^R, respectively. This agent acts by blocking the enzyme that promotes intestinal absorption of dietary fat. Being relatively safe, it is moderately effective as an adjunct to dieting, but if one consumes meals with prominent fat content, it may produce excessive gas, diarrhea, and involuntary discharge of stool (you may want to avoid parties!). Moreover, it may interfere with the absorption of several fat soluble medications and vitamins A, D, E, and K. Rarely liver damage can occur.

The second drug is Belviq[R] (lorcaserin), which promotes weight loss, apparently by increasing the brain's sensation of stomach fullness. In tests, this drug caused a modest weight loss averaging of 6 pounds in the first year, but after a second year most individuals gained back about a quarter of this meager amount. Side effects were common, including headaches, dizziness, fatigue, nausea, constipation, memory and attention problems, and, rarely, a leaky heart valve. Belviq can also interact with other drugs; therefore, one must pay close attention to all combinations.

The third drug is Qsymia (phentermine/topiramate), which is actually a combination of two medications—the stimulant phentermine and the antiseizure drug topiramate. Some trial participants lost as much as 10% of their body weight on this agent, but side effects were significant, including palpitations, reduction of memory and attention, problems with speech, anxiety, insomnia, and depression. Side effects were so prominent that about 40% of trial participants stopped taking it.

The fourth drug is Contrave[R] (naltrexone/bupropion), which seems to reduce appetite and cravings, again probably resulting from its effect on the brain. Small weight losses were recorded in those taking the drug, but fairly common were the side effects of nausea, constipation, headache, vomiting, dizziness, insomnia, dry mouth, and diarrhea.

Bottom Line

These drugs are not very "appetizing," and for most of us, they are best avoided. My own take is that the first drug, orlistat, might be the safest and probably the most effective of the group, but certainly not a real champion.

Last But Certainly Not Least: Surgery

For those who are severely obese, with a BMI of 40 or more, or those with a BMI above 35 with a serious health condition such as type 2 diabetes, surgical procedures can provide an effective last resort for weight reduction. Currently there are four types of procedures, all of which are designed to reduce the volume of the stomach in order to produce early satiation. All these procedures result in effective weight reductions but sometimes at a hefty cost, with somewhat high procedural risks. Resulting side effects may include diarrhea, cramps, stomach ulcers and bowel obstruction, provided that one survives the initial procedure. Nevertheless, if one is severely obese, one of these procedures may be quite helpful in achieving long-term weight reduction and reduction of presence and complications of diabetes, which is commonly associated with such massive overweight.

Conclusion:

If you can do it, stick to dieting!

ᶜᵍᐟᵖCHAPTER 2ᵉ⸾⸝

Eat a Good Breakfast: Was Mother Right or Wrong?

We have, from time immemorial, been universally admonished by mothers to eat a good breakfast. But why is this? Scientific information seems to be mixed—or at best inconclusive—about this matter. The 2010 Dietary Guidelines for Americans recommended breakfast for children but provided no guidance for adults, stating, "Behaviors have been studied, such as snacking or frequency of eating, but there is currently not enough evidence to support a specific recommendation for these behaviors." Results from a 2002 National Health and Nutrition Survey indicate that snacking and skipping breakfast are common, with 18% of the populace skipping breakfast and 86% snacking each day. Moreover, another US survey from 1965 to 1991 disclosed that, during that period, breakfast consumption had dropped from 86% to 75%. Thus, mothers seem to have lost control of sizeable portions of our population, exposing us to potentially risky eating habits.

Various small scientific studies have suggested that skipping breakfast may carry several adverse consequences, including weight gain, elevated blood cholesterol, high blood pressure, development of diabetes, and increased risk of heart disease. Although we can correlate skipping breakfast with various unfavorable outcomes, that does not prove a cause and effect relationship between the two. That is, do people who skip breakfast possess other traits such as intermittent snacking that predispose them to these various health risks? And would merely adding breakfast to one's ordinary eating habits produce the universal health benefits we desire?

Although still not conclusive, the evidence supporting the health benefits of eating breakfast in the long run continues to mount. A recent large study appearing in the American Heart Association Journal[4] showed that, after being followed for a period of 16 years, men who skipped breakfast had a 27% higher risk of heart disease compared with those who did not. What was most surprising about this study, however, was that, even though those skipping breakfast possessed more risk factors for cardiovascular diseases such as obesity, hypertension and diabetes, when the researchers corrected for these variables, those eating breakfast still had better long-term reductions of heart disease. This is powerful information that supports the idea that, by just including breakfast alone in your diet you may be reducing your chances of disease.

Some of the immediate benefits of breakfast are scientifically documented: These include improved concentration and performance at school or work, better physical strength, endurance, and improved eye-hand coordination. For simple weight reduction, however, short term omission of breakfast[5] (six weeks or less) fails to show much effect on weight, although those who eat breakfast tend to be more active and burn more calories shortly after this meal.

Another possibility contributing to the dangers of skipping breakfast is that, after an overnight fast, the body's metabolic rate slows sufficiently to slow the burning of calories, and by prolonging this fasting period, we are more apt to turn the furnace down to "low", burn up fewer calories, and allow for more conversion to fat that was designed for storage during lean periods. Despite the logic of this hypothesis, studies have been conflicting regarding its validity[6].

The longer term benefits of breakfast seem to be based on multiple factors as noted: Breakfast is more apt to contain more nutritious foods such as fruit and protein. Protein also provides more persistent satiation that delays hunger and, therefore, the desire for mid-morning snacks. Protein is especially helpful, for it not only provides a lengthier sense of fullness but also burns up more energy while being digested, resulting in fewer excess net calories to deal with. Therefore, don't forget to include protein sources such as eggs, yogurt, low-fat milk, cheese, nuts, etc., but minimize such processed meat sources as bacon, sausage and the like, for the latter pose, in themselves, significant threats to health (see chapter 17).

Conclusion:

I must admit that science—while moving at a fairly decent pace—has still not caught up with mother! So I say to one and all, eat your breakfast every morning, and it better be more than just a doughnut and coffee, or I'll tell mother on you!

⌒✐CHAPTER 3✑⌒

Trans Fat Consumption and Health

For the past several years, we have known that the so-called "trans fats" are unhealthy, but most people have little knowledge about these "little devils," how they threaten us, or how we can avoid them. I am prompted now by a recent study that has shown that, in this country at least, consumption continues at an excessively high rate.

The study to which I refer is entitled, "Trans fats still weighing Americans down," published by the American Heart Association[7]. The report began with "good news, bad news" that is, the amount of trans fats we eat has declined over the last 30 years, but we're still consuming more than recommended. In a study of over 12,000 adults 25-74 years of age, the results showed the following:

Trans fat intake dropped by about one–third in both men and women.

Average intake of the good omega–3 fatty acids (such as that derived from fish) was steady, but current intake was still very low.

Intake of saturated (bad) fats dropped, but still account for about 11.4 percent of daily calories for men and women.

The American Heart Association recommends limiting saturated fat to 5–6 percent of total calories.

The study disclosed that men consumed about 1.9 percent of their daily calories from trans fats and women about 1.7 percent. The American Heart Association recommends limiting trans fats to no more than 1 percent of total calories consumed, but ideally zero.

So let's take a closer look at this problem and see what we can do about it.

Trans fat is considered by most of the medical profession to be the worst type of fat consumed. Unlike other dietary fats, trans fat—also called trans-fatty acids—both raises your LDL ("bad") cholesterol and lowers your HDL ("good") cholesterol, and that spells "double trouble," because this combination poses a special risk of developing hardening of all the major arteries, increasing your risk of heart disease, which is the leading killer of both men and women. So, here's some information about trans fats and how to avoid them.

Most trans fats are formed through an industrial process that adds hydrogen to vegetable oil, causing the oil to become solid at room temperature. This manufactured form of trans fat bears the common name partially hydrogenated oil, which is convenient to use in margarine spreads and less likely to spoil, allowing foods made with it have a longer shelf life. Some restaurants even use this product in their deep fryers, because it doesn't have to be changed as often as do other oils. Although some meat and dairy products contain small amounts of naturally occurring trans fat, most of the latter are created in this manufactured form, found in the products noted below:

Baked goods: Most cakes, cookies, pie crusts, and crackers contain shortening, which is usually made from partially hydrogenated vegetable oil. Ready-made frosting is another source of trans fat.

Snacks: Potato, corn, and tortilla chips often contain trans fat. And while popcorn can be a healthy snack, many types of packaged or microwave popcorn use trans fat to help cook or flavor the popcorn.

Fried food: Foods that require deep frying—French fries, doughnuts, and fried chicken can contain trans fat from the oil used in the cooking process.

Refrigerator dough: Products such as canned biscuits and cinnamon rolls often contain trans fat, as do frozen pizza crusts.

Creamer and margarine: Nondairy coffee creamer and stick margarines also may contain partially hydrogenated vegetable oils.

So we are inundated by these devils, and this requires much diligence to reduce our intake. The American Heart Association recommends maximum reduction of foods containing trans fats. Reading and understanding the food labels is critical, because, in the United States, if a food has less than 0.5 grams of trans fat in a serving, its label can read 0 grams trans fat. This hidden trans fat can add up quickly, especially if you eat several servings of multiple foods containing less than 0.5 grams a serving. Therefore, when you check the label for trans fat, also check the food's ingredient list for partially hydrogenated vegetable oil—which indicates that the food contains some trans fat, even if the amount is below 0.5 grams. Even if a food is clearly free of trans fat, it is not automatically healthy. Food manufacturers have begun substituting other ingredients for trans fat. Some of these ingredients, such as tropical oils—coconut and palm oils— contain much saturated fat, which also raises your LDL cholesterol.

In a healthy diet, up to 25 to 35 percent of your total daily calories can come from fat—but saturated fat should account for less than 10 percent of your total daily calories. This usually involves preparing lean meats and poultry without added saturated and trans fats

Healthy Alternatives to Trans Fats

Monounsaturated fat—found in olive, peanut and canola oils—is a healthier option than is saturated or trans fat (see chapters 11 and 12). Nuts, fish and other foods containing unsaturated omega-3 fatty acids are other good choices of foods with monounsaturated fats.

After you study the labels carefully, adequate reduction of your trans fat intake will probably result in your cutting back all those snack food goodies that you desperately desire, even if your waistline doesn't.

But limiting these fats requires more than individual effort, since we are still at the mercy of restaurants and other public food sources, and this generally requires legislative action. Until recently, retail food establishments were exempt from federal nutrition labeling requirements, so consumers had no consistent way of determining which restaurant foods contain high levels of artificial trans fat, and thus no practical means of avoiding them. Interestingly, the much maligned Affordable Care Act, passed in 2010, is helping to change that situation. This law includes a menu labeling law which requires retail food establishments to disclose calorie information on their menus, and to make other nutritional information, including trans fat content, available in written form to consumers upon request, and prior to purchase. The Food & Drug Administration is in the process of finalizing the regulations to implement the law.

Additional efforts to eliminate artificial trans fat from foods have gained momentum. In 2012, the USDA issued final rules for the national school breakfast and lunch programs, which added a requirement that food products and ingredients used to make these meals contain less than .5 gm added trans fat per serving. A number of states and localities also have considered legislative proposals to limit or eliminate artificial trans fat use in food service establishments. To date, trans fat bans have passed in roughly a dozen localities including New York City, and one state— California—has imposed a statewide ban on artificial trans fat in restaurants. Legislation banning the use of artificial trans fats in restaurants has gained currency across the United States. This battle, however, is far from over, since legal challenges are likely to arise from near and far.

CHAPTER 4

Coffee and Health: Good, Bad, or Indifferent?

Second only to water, coffee is the most widely consumed beverage in the United States. Approximately two thirds of American adults drink coffee, consuming more than 400 million cups daily, a total that exceeds every other individual nation. For this reason, we must constantly monitor this beverage for any possible ill effects it may have on health. This issue has been carefully reviewed in a recent study[8]. Although caffeine is the main component, coffee contains hundreds of biologically active compounds that could play a potential role in human health.

The study noted above found that coffee exerts mixed effects on overall health, but, on balance, it does not produce adverse outcomes. The potentially beneficial effects from coffee are a modest reduction of the incidence of type 2 diabetes, hypertension (high blood pressure), obesity, and depression. Moreover, habitual coffee consumption either has no effect or is modestly beneficial for prevention of heart disease and stroke.

Overall mortality—from both cardiovascular and other causes—seems to be favorably influenced by coffee consumption. Benefits from coffee seem to stem from better asthma control and a lower risk of certain neurologic and gastrointestinal disorders. On the other hand, certain risks of coffee consumption are attributable primarily to its caffeine content. These include anxiety, insomnia, tremulousness, and palpitations. There also is a possible increased risk of bone loss and fractures. Moreover, coffee prepared by boiling appears to raise levels of cholesterol in the blood, whereas filtered coffee lacks this effect. Whether these latter differences make a difference in long-term outlook are unclear.

So, overall, coffee seems to receive a reasonably clean bill of health, provided it is not consumed in excess. The upper limit of safe consumption is not clearly established, but approximately 2-3 cups per day, preferably by the process of filtration, appears to be safe and attended by neutral to beneficial effects. Or at least it does not seem to pose any real risk to health or longevity.

CHAPTER 5

Green Tea: Possible Health Benefits

Tea, especially green tea, or camellia sinensi, is a rich source of flavonols, compounds that seem to benefit cardiovascular health. Flavonols are widely present not only in green tea, but also in cocoa, red wine, and some fruits. The most abundant and most active flavonol in green tea is epigallocatechin gallate, and it likely has the greatest potentially beneficial effects. Among these benefits is enhanced control of blood sugar levels through improvement of insulin utilization by the body. Other advantages include decreased cholesterol absorption from the intestines and the lowering of blood pressure levels.

Recent studies[9,10] have evaluated the published information on the effects of green tea and its extract on blood pressure, cardiovascular disease development, and blood sugar control in both diabetics and non-diabetics. The researchers found that green tea consumption significantly reduced the incidence and complications of cardiovascular disease, and helped to reduce blood sugar levels, contributing to better management of the diabetic state. Moreover, green tea intake results in significant reductions in blood pressure, total cholesterol, and LDL (bad) cholesterol. The effect on blood pressure was small, but the effects on total and LDL cholesterol were moderate. Black tea exhibits similar, although lesser, effects.

Since diabetes is quite common and is a serious threat to health, green tea could play a role in both prevention and management of this disorder. In addition to changes in life style (proper diet, weight reduction, and exercise), regular consumption of green tea might be a useful adjunct.

So how much green tea should one consume to reduce disease development and blood sugar levels? The available data suggest that, in comparison with non-tea drinkers, the benefits progressively increase with tea consumption increasing from one to greater than four cups daily. But since it's a matter of taste, green tea may not be for everyone. If you like this product, however, especially if you are diabetic or at risk for later development of cardiovascular disease, consider regular consumption of green tea—unsweetened of course.

ᴄ⁄᭒CHAPTER 6᭒

Chocolate: Is it Really Good for What Ails You?

Now it May Even Help the Brain Function

I n recent years much has been written about the health value of dark chocolate. Chocolate contains a class of flavanols, which, as already noted, are widely present in cocoa, green tea, red wine, and some fruits. These components seem to be helpful in lowering blood pressure and improving cardiovascular health. Recent research has suggested that they can even provide a boost to brain function, wherein it seemed to slow the progression of mental decline that occurs with aging[11]. Although this concept seems somewhat tentative—to say the least—now a seemingly more audacious assertion states that populations that consume more chocolate also produce per capita the most Nobel laureates. Correlating the per capita chocolate consumption, Messerli[12] found a strong relationship across numerous countries. China scored lowest, and Switzerland, highest, in this category. The U.S.A. scored midway between these two extremes.

But even though a correlation exists between chocolate and apparent brain function, this does not necessarily mean that chocolate causes the brain to work better. Other factors could account for this relationship. For instance, more affluent societies that provide higher levels of education might also possess the financial resources to purchase more chocolate. But the idea that chocolate can produce such a far-out effect is thought provoking, and worthy of more structured research, especially considering that chocolate seems to enhance general cardiovascular health and probably increases blood flow to the brain.

But let's also take a closer look at chocolate, for the story is not uniformly rosy: Unconstrained consumption of large quantities of chocolate, without a corresponding increase in activity, increases the risk of obesity. Raw chocolate is high in cocoa butter, a high-caloric fat removed during chocolate refining, then added back in varying proportions during manufacturing. Manufacturers may add other fats, sugars, and milk as well, all of which increase the caloric content of chocolate.

Limited research indicates that cocoa or dark chocolate may produce certain beneficial effects on human health. In test tubes, cocoa has antioxidant activity, an effect highly doubtful in relation to the living human body. Some studies have also observed that those consuming dark chocolate daily experience a modest reduction in blood pressure with dilation of arteries, resulting in increased circulation to various organs (the brain for one, as noted above). Consuming milk chocolate or white chocolate, or drinking fat-containing milk with dark chocolate, appears to largely negate this beneficial effect.

Although the findings are limited, one study found that survivors of heart attacks who ate chocolate at least two or three times a week reduced their risk of death by a factor of up to threefold, compared to survivors who did not eat chocolate. These apparently beneficial effects have been confirmed in more recent reviews, supporting the positive role of cacao and cocoa products on cardiovascular risk factors such as blood pressure, cholesterol levels, atherosclerosis, and improving how the body handles insulin (potentially helping diabetes, another potent risk factor).

A recent large review[13] of pooled research data also strongly pointed toward a beneficial role for chocolate. Although this review reiterated the fact that over-consumption can have harmful effects, the existing studies generally agree that chocolate consumption might lower the risk of cardiovascular disorders, including heart attacks (myocardial infarctions), strokes, and even diabetes. These authors warned, however, that corroboration of this relationship is now required from additional studies, especially prospective experimental studies to test causation rather than just association between chocolate and disease.

How should the individual react to this information? Considering the limited data available, we must counsel caution. Nevertheless, the current evidence suggests that chocolate might be helpful in the prevention of cardiovascular disorders if consumed in moderation, especially if efforts are made to reduce the sugar and fat content of currently available products. One should be careful, therefore, to check the labeling of contents of the existing products. We also don't really know how much consumption of any of these products might be helpful. The European Union Commission recently approved a health claim that 200 milligrams of cocoa flavanols can "help maintain the elasticity of blood vessels, which contributes to normal blood flow." This daily dose is equivalent to 2.5 grams (about half teaspoonful) of high-flavanol dark chocolate (about one fifth of a regular size chocolate bar).

Conclusion:

Since most people like chocolate—I, for one—and if you can take it regularly without gaining weight, it certainly should do no harm! Maybe we should consider substituting hot chocolate for coffee, at least some of the time.

CHAPTER 7

Some Foods to Avoid

Previously I had suggested several foods to be included in healthy diets. In this communication, I list an "all-star" cast of some foods that should be strenuously avoided. Representing merely examples, these instances are blatant offenders and constitute only the "tip of the iceberg" of nefarious foods. And we wonder why we have such an epidemic of obesity, heart attacks, and high blood pressure here and in so many other parts of the world!

1. Chicken Pot Pie. As an example, Marie Callender's pie, while presumably tasty, contains 22 grams of saturated fat, 1,600 mg of sodium, and possesses "only" 1,040 calories. I suspect that most such pies will be equally dangerous. Check them out first, or stay away entirely.

2. Parkay Margarine sticks. They may be cholesterol-free, but each tablespoon of the spread has 1.5 grams of undesirable trans-fat and an equal amount of equally undesirable saturated fat. Other similar products are just as deadly, i.e., Blue Bonnet, Land O'Lakes, Country Crock, and Fleischmann's. Instead of

these stick margarines, look for tub margarines instead, for most have little or no trans-fat.

3.   Canned Soups: As an example, an average cup of Campbell's regular Condensed Soup contains up to 1,900 mg of sodium in a single can (supposedly two servings, but many will opt for the whole can)—more than most adults should consume in an entire day! For more on sodium, see chapters 13 and 14. For best results, look for Campbell's Healthy Choice soups containing around 400 mg of sodium (which is still a bit too much). Other standard brands also contain loads of salt. To minimize these amounts, I suggest reduced-sodium soups by Amy's, Imagine Foods, Pacific Natural Foods, Dr. McDougall's light sodium, and Tabatchnick.

4.   Tortillas: For instance, Chipoltle Chicken Burrito (tortilla, rice, pinto beans, cheese, chicken, sour cream, and salsa) contains 970 calories, 18 grams of saturated fat, and 2,200 mg of sodium. Skipping the cheese and sour cream cuts the saturated fat to 6 grams, but the remaining bulk contains more than a day's worth of sodium. Not my recommendation.

5.   Desserts with a Vengeance: How about Cheesecake Factory's Chocolate Tower Truffle Cake for a winner! This slab of cake weighs 3/4 lb, containing 1,760 calories with 50 grams of saturated fat, which. I would call a deadly dish.

6.   Biscuits that are far from healthy: Try Pillsbury Grands! Each one of these southern style frozen biscuits has 170 calories and 1 1/2 grams of trans fat. While other companies are dumping their partially hydrogenated oils (trans fats), Pillsbury still makes most of its rolls and biscuits with this nasty stuff.

7.　　　Not so Mediterranean: This dish has a misleading name, so don't go near Olive Garden's "Tour of Italy", which consists of homemade lasagna, lightly breaded chicken Parmigiana, and creamy fettuccine alfredo. It contains 1,450 calories, 33 grams of saturated fat, and 3,830 milligrams of sodium. If you add a breadstick (150 calories and 400 mg of sodium) with a garden salad with dressing (290 calories and 1,530 mg of sodium), you'll be well on your way to needing heart bypass surgery. Although I am capable of treating heart disease, I much prefer preventing it.

8.　　　Starbucks gets into the act: The Starbucks Venti (20oz) White Chocolate Mocha with 2% milk and whipped cream is more than a simple cup of coffee. It possesses 580 calories, 14 grams of saturated fat, and 13 teaspoons of added sugar. You can, however, minimize the damage by 130 calories and cut the saturated fat in half if you order it with nonfat milk and no whipped cream.

9.　　　Ice cream is no bargain: An average half cup serving of plain vanilla Haagen-Dazs ice cream contains about 250 calories, but, unfortunately, 10 grams of undesirable saturated fat. And that's only if you don't add any toppings or whipped cream. Of all the threatening foods on this page, this may be the lesser of the evils.

10.　　　A loaded milk shake: Cold Stone Creamery's "Oh Fudge" shake contains chocolate ice cream, milk, and fudge syrup, starting at 1,060 calories for the small "Like It" (16 oz.) size. It becomes progressively worse with the medium "Love it" (20 oz.), with 1,360 calories, and the large "Gotta Have It" (24 oz.), with 1,600 calories and 62 grams of saturated fat. That's the saturated fat content of two 16 oz. rib eye steaks plus a buttered baked potato. I suppose if you're running marathons every few days, you could handle this much caloric load, provided you don't drop dead in the process.

Hopefully, I haven't spoiled your entire day by advising against such yummy foods. But even if your day is less fun, your future has a chance to be much more secure and probably substantially longer.

⊂≪CHAPTER 8≫⊃

Do Cranberries Deserve Top Billing Over Turkey at Thanksgiving?

According to a recent analysis, cranberries and their juice may substantially reduce the risk for urinary tract infections. Pooled quantitative data from nine trials, including 1175 individuals, showed that cranberry consumption could reduce the risk for these infections by 38% overall and by 51% in women[14].

"Cranberry-containing products tend to be more effective in women with recurrent urinary tract infections, children, cranberry juice drinkers, and people using cranberry-containing products more than twice daily," say Chien-Chang Lee (National Taiwan University Hospital) and colleagues.

In the 9 studies that assessed cumulative incidence of such infections, final analysis showed that, as well as reducing the risk for infections in the population as a whole, cranberry consumption also helped prevention in women with recurrent urinary infections, reducing their risk by 47%. In most of the studies, participants took the products for 6 months.

Men generally don't suffer from such problems, except in old age. By contrast, 40-50% of women will experience at least one urinary tract infection during their lifetime, of which 20-30% will become recurrent.

The review disclosed that cranberry juice was more effective than cranberry capsules or tablets. This could be due to better hydration in those taking juice, or that there might be an unidentified substance within cranberry juice that is not found in cranberry capsules. Capsules may be more appropriate, however, for diabetics in order to avoid excess sugar or calories.

Although the mechanism by which cranberry consumption can prevent such infections is unclear, proanthocyanidin, found in cranberries, has been found to prevent the adherence of the bacteria, Escherichia coli, to the urinary tract lining. Or it may simply result from acidification, and/or increased volume, of urine resulting from such juice, providing a less favorable environment for bacterial growth.

The authors concluded: "The results of the present meta-analysis support that consumption of cranberry-containing products may protect against infections in certain populations. However, because of the substantial heterogeneity across trials, this conclusion should be interpreted with great caution." They also call for more dose-response studies to determine optimal dosing. One such study is currently underway.

But the probable benefits of cranberries don't end here: The National Institutes of Health is funding research on cranberry's effects on heart disease, various infections, and other conditions, and other researchers are investigating its potential against cancer, stroke, and viruses.

So far, research has disclosed:

The proanthocyanidine in cranberries prevents plaque formation on teeth; mouthwashes containing it are being developed to prevent periodontal disease.

In some people, regular cranberry juice consumption for months can kill the H. pylori bacteria, which can cause stomach cancer and ulcers.

Preliminary research also shows:

Drinking cranberry juice daily may increase levels of HDL, or good cholesterol, and reduce levels of LDL, or bad cholesterol.

Cranberries may prevent some tumors from growing rapidly or starting in the first place. For instance, extracts of chemicals in cranberries prevent breast cancer cells from multiplying in a test tube; whether that would work in women is unknown.

The Bottom Line?

Since cranberry juice is nutritious and safe, why not drink two or more glasses a day, especially if you are a woman at risk for urinary infections (and maybe breast cancer?) So try to include cranberries and sauce in meals extending beyond Thanksgiving. There is no harm in this strategy, even before more definitive information is available.

I assure the reader I have no conflicting financial interest in the cranberry industry.

⋐⋗CHAPTER 9⋐⋗

Fish Consumption: Some Safety Issues

Fish consumption is heart-healthy and provides an excellent source of protein. But there are certain associated risks. One of these is the fact that fish may contain mercury, which is a well-known toxin. When consumed in excess, mercury can cause damage to brain and nervous system causing prickly sensations with various additional problems with fine muscular coordination, speech, sleep, and walking. At highest risk are pregnant women and young children.

Unfortunately, many fish species do contain mercury, which is consumed from plants and tiny animals. When smaller fish are then eaten by larger fish, the latter's tissue accumulates increasing amounts of mercury. Thus larger, predatory fish such as sharks and swordfish generally contain more mercury than smaller fish such as sardines, sole, and trout. Compounding this problem, mercury levels in the northern Pacific Ocean have risen about 30% over the past 20 years and are expected to rise further because of industrial input.

If you want to consume fish (and you should), here are my suggestions:

Consume the lowest mercury fish, which are the following: Wild and Alaska salmon, sardines, tilapia, and shellfish such as shrimp, scallops, oysters, and squid.

Still low, but slightly higher, are haddock, flounder, sole, catfish, trout, codfish, and Atlantic mackerel.

The highest ones, to be generally limited or avoided, are swordfish, shark, king mackerel, orange roughy, marlin, grouper, Chilean sea bass, bluefish, halibut, Spanish mackerel (Gulf), and fresh or canned tuna.

The FDA and EPA warn most women (especially if pregnant) and children, against consumption of those fish in the highest mercury group noted above. Moreover, if you are a frequent consumer of more than 24 ounces of any type of fish each week, you are advised to avoid this latter category as much as possible.

Guidelines for limits on fish consumption are undergoing continued scrutiny.

Conclusion:

Women who are of childbearing age should limit themselves to no more than 12 ounces per week, primarily consuming those fish groups having the lowest mercury content. Similar limitations should be applied to children. As noted above, adults should limit their intake of high-mercury types of fish.

A useful tool to provide safer and more specific seafood choices can be found at Consumer Reports website: ConsumerReports.org/org/cro/mercury1014. You can enter the types and amounts of fish you plan to consume, along with your body weight, and you will know whether you'll be within acceptable limits.

CHAPTER 10

Shellfish: Nutrition and Health

A re shellfish as healthy as regular fish?

In general, fish (such as baked salmon) is a very healthy food choice, containing beneficial proteins and omega-3 fats. As noted in chapter 9, you'd best go light on swordfish and other species known to contain mercury, but otherwise, no real limitations. But is the same true for shellfish such as lobster, shrimp, or clams?

To answer that question, the Department of Agriculture's nutrient database contains some important advice:

Omega-3s and Shellfish

If you're eating cold-water fish like salmon because of the beneficial omega-3s, then shellfish may not be a great substitute. Lobster contains very few omega-3s, and shrimp and clams are pretty modest contributors. Calamari, blue crab, and oysters have about a fourth of the omega-3 content of salmon, or about as much as a fish like flounder, which isn't bad at all.

Regarding protein content, ounce for ounce, all shellfish are pretty much in the same neighborhood as salmon (clams are a bit on the low side). But if you are really serious about protein, eat some octopus, which contains more protein than most species of fish.

Cholesterol

Ingested saturated fat has a bigger effect on our blood cholesterol levels than the cholesterol we eat. Still, some people are "cholesterol responders"—meaning the amount of cholesterol they eat greatly impacts their blood cholesterol levels. For them, a steady diet of shrimp (which has 166 mg. of cholesterol per 3 ounces) and fried calamari (221 mg.) might present a problem.

But clams, crab, mussels, and oysters tend to lower cholesterol levels a little bit, partly because they contain compounds called sterols that interfere with the absorption of cholesterol.

Calorie Content

Naturally, the calorie count goes up for anything that's breaded and fried. But the good news: shellfish are low in calories.

Nutritional Advantages

Shellfish contain some components not well understood. Oysters are an excellent source of zinc. Clams contain a lot of iron and vitamin B12. And crustaceans are champion suppliers of choline, an obscure nutrient that accelerates the synthesis of acetylcholine, a neurotransmitter important in memory and muscle control.

On the other hand, stay away from jellyfish. Nutritionally they have little to offer. The dried, salted jellyfish listed in the nutrient database contains a great amount of sodium, and there's far too much of it already.

Toxins

There are other issues with shellfish besides nutritional pros and cons. Toxins can be a problem. The reddish-brown organisms called dinoflagellates that are responsible for "red tides" make a toxin that collects in many different species, including clams, crabs, mussels, and scallops. In 2008, the FDA put out an advisory telling people not to eat tomalley, the soft green substance in lobster, because of red-tide conditions.

If you eat shellfish containing high concentrations of the red-tide toxin, you could come down with a case of paralytic shellfish poisoning. This scary-sounding disease can be deadly, but the symptoms of paralytic shellfish poisoning are usually mild. They include numbness and tingling sensations that may be followed by a headache, dizziness, or a strange floating sensation.

Another type of dinoflagellate produces a different toxin that causes a condition called neurotoxic shellfish poisoning. And a species of microscopic algae called Pseudo-nitzschia produces a toxin that causes a third condition, amnesic shellfish poisoning. About 30 cases of poisoning by marine toxins (shellfish and finfish combined) are reported each year in the United States, and it's possible that many minor cases go unreported. One death occurs, on average, every four years. Still, getting sick from toxin-laden shellfish is a rare event. You should, though, keep an eye out for health advisories about red tides and other toxin-generating "blooms" and eat accordingly.

Allergies

People also occasionally get sick from eating shellfish because of allergies. About 2% of adult Americans are believed to have food allergies, and allergies to shellfish are among the most common. The reactions vary, but they can be rather severe. There are case reports in the medical journals of shellfish causing anaphylactic shock and even a small number of deaths. Some people are allergic to differing types of shellfish, with considerable overlap between species. As a practical matter, people who are allergic to one type of shellfish are best advised to avoid them all.

CHAPTER 11

Some Foods are Better Than You May Think

We have always known about the general benefit of adding all fruits and vegetables to the diet for overall health. They should be part of our everyday consumption. Surprisingly good health perks are at your fingertips in your own refrigerator or pantry. Let's look at a few and note their benefits.

1. Red Bell Pepper: One cup of chopped red bell pepper has more than twice the amount of vitamin C than a medium-sized orange. So, even if your regular diet contains adequate amounts of this vitamin (which may or may not help support your immune system), if you add in a few peppers, there is no need to worry about taking supplemental vitamin C.

2. Potatoes: Often maligned because of their high carbohydrate content, purple and white potatoes are rich in both magnesium and potassium. According to recent evidence, these two minerals can lower the risk of hypertension (high blood pressure), which is a very common affliction in our society.

3. Raspberries: A cup of raspberries contains a hefty amount (8 grams) of beneficial fiber, which can aid in better hunger satiation and digestive

function. This amount of fiber more than doubles that found in a cup of apple slices.

4. Peas: These veggies possess a surprisingly large content of protein, which builds and supports muscle tissue. One cup of peas contains 8 grams of protein, 2 grams more than you'll find in a large egg, and as an extra dividend, peas possess none of the cholesterol possessed by eggs.

More Berries and More Good News!

There is extra value provided by blueberries, strawberries, and other similar sources (eggplants, blackberries, and black currants). Evidence is beginning to support this contention, for the following results recently appeared in a leading medical journal sponsored by the American Heart Association[15]. Although the study was limited to young and middle aged women, the implications certainly extend beyond this group.

The researchers analyzed dietary data from 93,600 women enrolled in the Nurses' Health Study II to determine the effect of dietary flavanoids, which are known to benefit blood vessel function, on health outcomes. The study covered nearly 20 years, and researchers concluded that those who consume high levels of anthocyanins—the flavonoids present in red and blue fruits such as strawberries and blueberries—had a significantly reduced risk for heart attacks (myocardial infarctions). The analysis showed that women who consumed three servings of strawberries or blueberries weekly had a 34% decrease in risk of this heart affliction compared with women who rarely included these fruits in their diet.

Furthermore, when the researchers looked at the sliding scale relating those consuming the greatest to the lowest amounts of these fruits, they noted the presence of a dose-response relationship, another important feature that helps us to establish a causative role for these dietary influences. This risk reduction persisted even when the researchers adjusted for total fruit and vegetable intake, suggesting "that the benefits are specific to a food constituent in anthocyanin-rich foods (including blueberries, strawberries, eggplants, blackberries, black currants), and not necessarily to nonspecific benefits among participants who consume high intakes of other fruits and vegetables."

However, the researchers noted that there may be other unidentified, potentially beneficial components in other fruits and vegetables that contribute to the protection that their population-based study was not powered to detect. They called for more research to better understand anthocyanins' mechanism of action in heart protection, as well as to further evaluate dose responses and longer-term clinical endpoints.

Now a more recent study[16] added further support to the benefits of berries, for high intake of blueberries and strawberries by older women appeared to delay cognitive aging by up to 2.5 years. Over a six year period, 16,000 women aged 70 or more were tested for memory and cognitive function. Their conclusion? Two or more weekly servings of blueberries and strawberries reduced memory decline as compared with those eating less.

Conclusion:

All of us should include these fruits (as well as the wider spectrum of fruits and vegetables) in our diets on a regular basis. What is less apparent from such research is also worth emphasizing: Taking supplemental vitamins—no matter how great in amount—will not provide the protection coming from the real thing, i.e. the food itself.

Beets and Juice

Beets are a good source of nutrition because they contain potassium, magnesium, iron, vitamins A, B6 and C, folic acid, carbohydrates, nitrates, protein, and soluble fiber.

But there are extra benefits to be had from consumption of this vegetable: They can even enhance athletic performance. Scientific studies[17] have shown that the nitrate found in beetroot concentrate increases blood flow to skeletal muscles during exercise. This forms the basis for how this juice may benefit football players by preferentially increasing blood flow to the so-called "fast–twitch" muscle fibers—the ones used for explosive running. Additional studies have shown that beetroot juice improved performance by 2.8% (11 seconds) in a 4-km bicycle time trial and by 2.7% (45 seconds) in 16.1-km time trial. For these reasons, the Auburn University football team revealed its pregame ritual of taking beet juice concentrate before each game. Perhaps this explains Auburn's football success of late!

But the benefits of beets go beyond sports to the general population. Researchers have long known that beet juice may help lower blood pressure. A 2008 study examined the effects of ingesting 500ml (1 pint) of beetroot juice in healthy volunteers and found that blood pressure was significantly lowered after ingestion. Additional study[18] has suggested that nitrate (converted to nitrite in the body) is likely the special component that lowers blood pressure and may help to fight heart disease. This finding should apply at least to people with very high blood pressure—who may require multiple tablets—to a more natural approach. Further support to this concept was provided by a more recent study by scientists from Queen Mary University of London[19], who found that drinking a daily cup of beetroot juice (8 oz.) significantly lowered blood pressure among hypertensive patients. They recorded an average decrease in blood pressure of about 8 mmHg (which for many patients brought their blood pressure levels back into the 'normal' range). This is due to beetroot—and other leafy green vegetables such as lettuce and cabbage—containing high nitrate levels. The potential importance of these findings is substantial because large-scale observational studies suggest that each 2mmHg increase in blood pressure increases the likelihood of death from heart disease by 7 per cent and stroke by 10 per cent. This was the first evidence of a long-lasting blood pressure reduction with dietary nitrate supplementation in a relevant patient group.

Because of these additional benefits, beets have been subject of much coverage in the media, being generally linked not only to lower blood pressure, but also to better stamina and improved blood flood throughout the body. How much of these latter claims are true, however, remains to be seen.

Nuts and Seeds: Health Effects As Good As Medicine?

Nuts

This category includes nuts from trees, including almonds, hazelnuts, walnuts, pistachios, pine nuts, cashews, pecans, macadamias, and Brazil nuts. Although not technically a "tree nut," peanuts possess similar traits and are, therefore, included in this category.

Most of these nuts provide good sources of caloric energy, primarily from unsaturated fats (oils), useful also for lowering cholesterol. Moreover, the essential amino acids contained in nuts are vital for constructing protein, i.e., the building blocks for our muscles and other tissues. Although each type of nut does not supply, in itself, a complete source of these amino acids, consuming a variety of nuts will provide a complete complement of the various necessary (essential) components. Other nutritional elements provided by nuts include folic acid, vitamin E, potassium, magnesium, and calcium. Especially noteworthy is their uniformly low sodium content, a highly desirable feature (provided that no salt is added). They also contain polyphenols, bioactive constituents that seem to be beneficial to heart health that extends beyond other dietary efforts.

During the past 20 years, mounting evidence indicates that consuming these nuts (including peanuts and peanut butter) at least twice weekly provides substantial protection from cardiovascular disease and overall death rates as compared to those consuming them only rarely or not at all[20,21]. These desirable results seem to be obtained primarily through the lowering of unfavorable cholesterol components, and despite a substantial caloric content, nuts have less tendency to promote obesity, probably because of their prominent satiating effect. For unknown reasons, nuts also appear to prevent diabetes, another contributor to cardiovascular disease. Research studies have also indicated that, if the "Mediterranean" diet, which, in itself is healthy, is supplemented by extra mixed nuts (one ounce daily) and extra virgin olive oil (one quart total per week), substantial additional reductions of cardiovascular disease and stroke can be accomplished.

Seeds

Edible seeds that contribute to human nutrition include grains (e.g. wheat, corn, rice, barley, millet, and oats), legumes (e.g. soybeans), cocoa and coffee beans. Some grains, however, are less beneficial, and these include white rice, white bread, pasta, noodles, and refined grain products with added sugar, fat, and sodium (e.g. biscuits, pastries, and cakes). Cocoa beans are the seeds of the tropical tree *Theobroma cacao*, from which chocolate is derived.

Whole grains comprise germ, bran, and endosperm. Refining them reduces their nutritional quality by removing beneficial constituents that include germ and bran along with fiber, vitamins minerals, phenolic compounds, and phytochemicals. Large studies have demonstrated a 21% lower risk of cardiovascular disease with greater longevity for those individuals consuming an average of 3-5 servings per day compared with those who rarely or never consumed whole grains. This group also had a 26% lower risk for the development of diabetes. In comparison to germ, bran seemed to be more potent in this regard.

Cocoa and chocolate require special comment. As noted previously, all research clearly confirms the value of chocolate in the prevention of cardiovascular disease, probably through improved cholesterol and blood pressure levels as well as reduced development of diabetes. Dark chocolate (as opposed to white or milk chocolate) is the most beneficial, but the effect of milk chocolate alone cannot be clearly established since many studies do not separate the two types for individual analysis.

Although seeds, nuts, and chocolate possess high fat content, it is polyunsaturated in type, which decreases cholesterol levels, metabolism of sugar (reducing diabetic tendency) and cardiovascular risk. Whole grains are rich in insoluble fiber (bran), a beneficial non-absorbable nutrient that, for unclear reasons, is also associated with reduced diabetes and cardiovascular risk

Pulses

"Pulses" are the seeds of plants contained within pods, and they include lentils, chickpeas, black-eyed peas, and a variety of beans that include pinto, kidney, navy, and fava beans.

Scientific studies regularly indicate that consumption of these food sources reduces the incidence of cardiovascular disease. One study demonstrated that their consumption four times weekly was associated with a 22% lower risk of heart disease in comparison with those who consumed them less than once weekly. Similar results are found when beans are substituted for white rice.

The beneficial effects of pulses seem to result primarily from their favorable effects on cholesterol components and enhancement of sugar metabolism that improves prevention and control of diabetes.

Conclusion:

In general, one should attempt to substitute whole grains and legumes for refined grains in all diets. Moderate consumption of cocoa products can be incorporated. Separating the effects of different components of seeds and nuts is not possible, and therefore, dietary recommendations should include a wide array of those foods listed earlier in this chapter as a major part of a plant-based diet. These modifications should be included with other components of a healthy diet that are well known, such as avoidance of red meat, reduction of salt intake, limitation of caloric intake, and regular inclusion of breakfast.

CHAPTER 12

Olive Oil and Health

O live oil contains monounsaturated fatty acids (MUFAs), which are considered a healthy dietary fat. If your diet replaces saturated and trans fats with unsaturated fats such as MUFAs and polyunsaturated fats (PUFAs), you may gain many health benefits. These fats may help lower your risk of cardiovascular disease by improving well-known risk factors such as lowering your total cholesterol and low-density lipoprotein (bad) cholesterol levels. MUFAs may also help normalize blood clotting. And some research shows that MUFAs may also benefit insulin levels and blood sugar control, which can be especially helpful if you have diabetes. Olive oil is recognized as one of the healthiest edible oils since it contains linoleic (omega-6) and linolenic acid (omega-3) essential fatty acids in favorable quantities.

But the story of olive oil gets even better: Researchers from Hunter College in New York discovered that oleocanthal, another component in olive oil, causes selective damage to cancer cells without harming healthy ones. Since the Mediterranean diet is known to be associated with a reduced risk of many kinds of cancer, olive oil could be a major contributor to this benefit.

Finally, olive oil is also a very good source of vitamin K; 100 g (about 3 oz.) provides about 50% of daily requirements of this vitamin, useful for blood clotting. Vitamin K also has a potential role in promoting bone growth. It also has a potential role in Alzheimer's disease patients by limiting damage of brain cells.

But even healthy fat such as olive oil is high in calories, so use it only in moderation. Choose foods such as olive oil in place of other fatty foods—particularly butter and stick margarine.

Adding further to this beneficial role of olive oil, a recent study involving mice demonstrated how this oil, with its mono-unsaturated fat, might team up with nuts and nitrate-rich vegetables such as spinach and celery, to produce chemical reactions that result in an enzyme that promotes blood-vessel dilation. This effect could potentially promote better circulation and defense against high blood pressure and other circulatory disorders. In addition, evidence also suggests that polyphenols in olive oil promote the main high density "good" lipoprotein (HDL), which promotes the body's elimination of the "bad" forms of cholesterol.

Bottom Line?

If not already doing so, you might consider using more liberal amounts of olive oil in your diet, especially in your salad dressings placed upon leafy greens, or on bread instead of butter. There is little reason not to.

CHAPTER 13

Sodium: Its Danger and Sneaky Ways It Enters Our Diets

The sodium we eat, mainly in the form of salt (sodium chloride), is a major cause of high blood pressure (hypertension)—a serious threat to health, usually accounting for premature death from cardiovascular disease. Salt, which is the main source of sodium, contains about 40% of this element. Hypertension affects almost 75 million American adults, rising to a lifetime probability for individuals with advancing age to as high as 90%. Although blood pressure can be controlled with medication, as many as 50% of individuals suffering from high blood pressure still remain above desirable levels despite such treatment. Even in those whose blood pressure is controlled with medication, their risk of developing heart disease and stroke remains higher than for those who have a normal blood pressure level naturally.

Studies uniformly show that cutting down on sodium (the primary component of table salt) in your diet can lower blood pressure—reducing your risk of stroke, heart failure and other health problems.

Although the exact numbers are still controversial, experts say most people should consume less than 2,300 mg of sodium each day. That's about the contents found in

1.5 teaspoon of table salt. People with certain medical conditions should consume even less.

The average American consumes at least 3,400 mg of sodium per day—or 48 percent or more than the recommended daily limit. So why is this? Unfortunately, huge amounts of sodium are unwittingly consumed when we dine in restaurants (chapter 14). But even at home we are subject to "sneaky" forms of sodium intake. For instance, one slice of white bread can contain as much as 230 mg. of sodium.

In the effort to seek a "healthier" form of salt, some believe that sea salt is the answer. No, it is not, for, although this latter form of salt is different in taste and texture, it contains the same amount of sodium as ordinary salt.

Avoiding the salt shaker is a useful start, but unfortunately, a major part of the sodium in American diets— almost 80 percent—comes from processed and packaged foods. These foods can be high in sodium even if they don't taste salty. They are summarized in the list below:

Summary of Sodium Levels Per 100 Gm (About 3 Oz) in Multiple Food Subcategories, in Descending Order.

Processed Foods (Per 100 Gm) Sodium

Food Milligrams

>Bacon (smoked) 1,803
>
>Salad Dressing, Caesar 1,079
>
>Barbecue Sauce, Original and Honey 989
>
>Hot Dogs 927
>
>Turkey Breast, sliced, Deli 878
>
>Macaroni and Cheese 831
>
>Pork Sausage 822

Cheese, Cheddar, sliced 645

Salsa, medium 611

Pizza, Pepperoni 560

Potato Chips and Crisps 547

Pizza, Cheese 521

Bread, White 500

Bread, Whole Wheat 493

Sauce, Spaghetti, tomato, marinara 407

Soup, Tomato 286

Tuna Fish, white, albacore, canned in water 261

Soup, Vegetable 243

Pork, Fresh or Frozen 186

Tomatoes, Canned, Diced 174

Chicken, Fresh or Frozen 77

RESTAURANT FOODS

Sausage Biscuits, breakfast 895

Chicken strips or tenders 736

Cheeseburgers, all sizes 568

Pizza, cheese, hand-tossed style 541

Grilled chicken sandwiches 525

French fries, medium 503

Hamburgers, all sizes 428

Checking labels is the only way to know how much sodium is in your food. If you buy packaged or processed foods, first choose foods that are labeled "sodium-free" or "very low sodium," but then check the actual numbers on the labels. Also, remember that the amount of sodium listed on the ingredient label references a particular serving size. If you eat more than the listed serving size, you'll consume more sodium.

Let's look at some ways to shop and cook low sodium:

Although we have provided a list above, let's review how much sodium is in popular foods.

The Centers for Disease Control has a list of six popular foods with high sodium content dubbed the "Salty Six."

1. Pizza – one slice can have up to 760 mg of sodium

2. Cold cuts and cured meats – Two slices of bologna

   a. can have 578 mg of sodium

   b. 3 Poultry – especially chicken nuggets. Just 3 ounces

   c. have nearly 600 mg of sodium

3. Canned soups – one cup of canned chicken noodle

   a. soup can have up to 940 mg of sodium

4. Sandwiches – consider the bread, cured meats,

   a. processed cheese and condiments, and sandwiches

   b. can easily surpass 1,500 mg of sodium

5. Breads and rolls – each piece can have up to 230 mg

   a. of sodium

Diet For High Blood Pressure

If you have high blood pressure, the DASH diet (Dietary Approaches to Stop Hypertension) is a low-sodium intervention that I present in chapter 16. Also good for the general population, most of the foods in that diet are also low in fat, and it includes four to five servings of fruit, four to five servings of vegetables, and two to three servings of low-fat dairy. It's also rich in whole grains, fish, poultry, beans, seeds, and nuts—while also limiting sugar and red meats.

Train Your Taste Buds

At first, foods may not taste as good without sodium. But you will adjust over time. Natural substitutes that taste great include lemon, ginger, curry, dried herbs (such as bay leaves, basil, and rosemary), onion, garlic, and dry mustard. You might also use salt substitutes, which are usually rich in beneficial potassium, but check with your doctor first, especially if you are taking any medications.

CHAPTER 14

More about Salt: Hidden Killer in Restaurant and Processed Foods

As I have noted in chapter 13, the sodium we eat, mainly in the form of salt is a major cause of high blood pressure With this background, the need for prevention and control of blood pressure is an urgent priority in this—and most other—nations. Although major lifestyle factors (avoiding obesity, regular exercise, moderation of alcohol intake, and diet rich in fruits, vegetables, and low fat dairy products) are important in reducing this risk, all the major health organizations have recognized sodium as the preeminent culprit and have recommended that each individual should control the amount of sodium he/she consumes, limiting it no more than 2,300 milligrams daily, and for high risk groups such as those with hypertension, diabetes, or chronic kidney disease, no more than 1,500 mg/day. No more than 1% of the population consumes as little as 1,500 mg/day. Although the media have expressed recent doubts about possible risks of consuming too little sodium, these doubts have been debunked by careful analysis[22].

According to one estimate, at least 150,000 premature deaths per year could be prevented in the U.S. alone if the sodium content of packaged and restaurant foods were reduced by 50%. This is especially meaningful since approximately 33% of calories are obtained from food purchased from restaurants and other sources outside of the home, constituting major and hidden sources of sodium. Overall, approximately 80% of the sodium consumed by Americans has been added by food manufacturers and restaurants. Are these latter companies doing anything to reduce this risk? The answer at present is very little, for one large survey[23] disclosed only minimal and inconsistent changes in the sodium content of their products—already far too high—between the years 2005 and 2011. To their credit, however, several major companies[24] have issued statements committing to lowering sodium levels in some products over the next several years. Especially noteworthy is that Walmart, the nation's largest supermarket chain, has called on its suppliers to lower sodium levels in their products by 25% by the year 2015. Nevertheless, even if these efforts are implemented, they would not nearly address the necessary reduction in sodium content. Thus short of a major public health initiative involving the federal government, we are unlikely to see sufficient voluntary changes in our food supply within the next several years.

So, given insufficient outside support, what can the individual do about this health danger? Urging the food industry voluntarily to label all ingredients contained in processed and restaurant foods would be a step in the right direction, but most are unlikely to do so unless they are forced. A public initiative directed at governmental leaders might also bring about some desired results in this direction. But, at present, limiting sodium intake is a matter of personal choice, and I have offered in chapter 13 some information about the contents of various processed and restaurant foods. But don't forget, adding any additional salt with the shaker amplifies the problem—so don't do it.

So at this time, all I can do is to wish everyone good luck in your food choices. Also remember to have your blood pressure checked at regular intervals, at least yearly, inasmuch as high blood pressure usually develops in the absence of warning symptoms or signs that might alert you to possible impending disaster.

CHAPTER 15

Potassium: A Great Dietary Constituent

Potassium is a dietary mineral necessary for many bodily functions. It plays an important role in holding blood pressure down, working in opposition to sodium. Potassium is also needed for normal muscle growth, and for nervous system and brain function. In addition to reducing blood pressure, potassium seems to work by protecting blood vessels from damage and excessive thickening. This mineral is found in many different foods, especially fruits and vegetables, so you may be getting plenty of potassium in your diet already. But for better understanding of your situation, we need to look at this issue more closely. Studies in human populations at risk for hypertension (high blood pressure) indicate that diets high in potassium can reduce the chances for this disorder with its devastating consequences, which includes strokes (brain damage), kidney failure, and heart disease. Although there is some debate regarding the optimal amount of dietary potassium, most authorities recommend a daily intake of at least 4,700 milligrams. Most Americans consume only half that amount per day, which would make them deficient in regards to this particular recommendation. Likewise, in the European Union, insufficient potassium intake is common. In a large pooled analysis, Italian researchers reported in 2011 that by raising one's daily intake of potassium by 1,640 milligram, you could expect a 21% lower risk of stroke. Even greater benefits can be achieved if we combine increased potassium with reduced intake of sodium.

In order to get 4,700 mg of potassium a day, try to get your intake from healthy eating unless your physician says otherwise. Dietary supplements containing potassium, while generally safe, can lead to excessive intake of this element that can be dangerous and, therefore, under most circumstances, are best avoided. Moreover, foods containing liberal amounts of potassium usually also possess other valuable nutrients that promote health in other ways. Several delicious foods can help you reach your potassium goal. Below is a list of great foods that can satisfy your needs as well as your eating pleasure.

1. Sweet potatoes: Surprisingly, this source outranks bananas on the list of foods that are high in potassium. One sweet potato packs a whopping 694 mg of potassium and only 131 calories, plus loads of fiber, beta-carotene (Vitamin A), and energizing carbohydrates. Baked, fried, grilled, mashed, or stuffed, sweet potatoes are one of the healthiest and most delicious foods you can eat. But be careful about what you put on them, avoiding large amounts of butter or trans fats.

2. Fresh tomatoes are great, but tomato paste and puree are even better sources of potassium. One quarter cup of tomato paste delivers 664 mg of this vital mineral, while one half cup of puree comes in at 549 mg. Tomato juice itself has just over 400 mg, but in general includes too much added sodium to be very beneficial. If you love cooking with tomatoes and want to get more potassium into your diet, make spaghetti sauce more often.

3.   Fresh beets: If you've ever bought fresh beets and tossed the greens in the garbage, time to change your ways. Those cooked, slightly bitter greens deserve a place at the table in part because they pack a whopping 644 mg of potassium per half cup. The beets themselves are also not only good for potassium (1 cup contains 440 mg) but they also provide generous amounts of folate (Vitamin B9), amounting to approximately 35% of daily adult requirements. Chapter 11 describes how beet juice may even enhance athletic performance.

4.   White beans are good providers of potassium, with half-a-cup delivering nearly 600 mg, but kidney and Lima beans, as well as lentils and split peas, are all respectable sources. All beans are good in general and appear prominently on our list of the best foods for fiber, so it's smart to make beans a much bigger part of your diet.

5.   Yogurt. Eight ounces of plain old non-fat yogurt contains 579 mg of potassium, while low-fat, whole milk, and cultured buttermilk—yogurt's tangy cousin—have a little less. Delicious ways to use yogurt include mixing it with granola at breakfast, using it instead of mayonnaise on sandwiches and in salads, and swapping it for whipped cream on desserts. Bonus: Most yogurt products contain probiotics, natural bacteria that can aid digestion and keep your gut healthy (Chapter 43).

6.   Clams: Canned or fresh, 3 ounces of clams pack 534 mg of potassium and have the highest concentration of vitamin B12 of any food. Use them to make seafood pasta or traditional New England clam chowder.

7.   Prunes: Juice from prunes is no joke when it comes to potassium, delivering 530 mg per 3/4 cup; half-a-cup of stewed prunes have nearly 400 mg. While you know prunes are good for regularity, you may not know that eating more of these dried plums can help keep your bones strong too. In one study, women who ate 10 prunes a day had significantly higher bone density than women who ate dried apples.

8.   Carrots: The juicing trend means more people will be getting their potassium from carrot juice, which packs over 500 mg in one 3/4 cup. Besides their potassium benefits, carrots and other orange-colored fruits and vegetables are also great for your eyes and vision.

9.   Molasses: Looking for a nutrient-packed alternative to sugar or honey? One tablespoon of blackstrap molasses (the thick, dark kind) has nearly 500 mg of potassium and a respectable amount of iron and calcium.

10.   Fish: Meaty fish like halibut and tuna have nearly 500 mg of potassium per 3 ounce serving, but cod and even farm-raised rainbow trout have plenty of potassium too. But potassium isn't the only reason to add more fish and seafood to your diet. Evidence is mounting that regularly eating fish, not taking fish supplements, can increase your lifespan, thanks in large part to the healthy fats in fresh fish; a high fish diet can even reduce your risk of death by heart disease by 35%, according to Harvard researchers.

11.   Soy: Unprocessed soy products (think edamame, not soy powder) are a great source of protein. One half cup of cooked soybeans contains nearly 500 mg of potassium.

12.   Squash: Winter squash like spaghetti squash are a dieter's dream: it contains less than 50 calories per serving, yet contains 448 mg of potassium per half cup. Also helpful is plenty of vitamin A and fiber.

13.   Bananas: Everyone thinks of bananas when they think of high-potassium foods, and one medium fruit does pack more than 400 mg of this mineral. But bananas are also the ultimate hunger buster, packed with healthy type of carbohydrate that is filling and tends to prevent subsequent hunger.

14.   Milk: This product is a surprising source of potassium, with 382 mg per cup for the non-fat or skim version (1% and whole milk contains a little less).

15.   Orange juice: One of the healthiest additions to your breakfast table is 3/4 of a cup of orange juice, which delivers 355 mg of potassium. Orange juice, especially the fresh-squeezed variety, is also a good source of calcium, folate, and several B vitamins.

So this list above can give you an idea of what foods to select with potassium in mind. But there are many more, too numerous to detail here. Below is a summary and more comprehensive list of foods that should be considered for inclusion in a healthy diet.

Foods High in Potassium:

Raisins

Prunes

Potatoes

Apricots

Dates

Strawberries

Bananas

Watermelon

Cantaloupe

Citrus fruits

Beets

Greens

Spinach

Tomatoes

Mushrooms

Soy and soy foods

Many veggie burgers

Peas

Beans

Turkey

Beef

Salmon

CHAPTER 16

Hypertension (High Blood Pressure) and The Dash Diet
What is Hypertension?

Hypertension is blood pressure that persistently stays higher than normal. Blood pressure is the force of blood against artery walls as the heart pumps blood through the body. Blood pressure can be unhealthy if it exceeds 140/90. (140 refers to the highest level reached with each heartbeat, and the 90, the low between these beats). The higher your blood pressure, the greater the health risk.

High blood pressure can be prevented or controlled if you take these steps:

1.   Maintain a healthy weight.

2.   Be physically active.

3.   Follow a healthy eating plan, which includes foods that do not contain a lot of salt (sodium), often referred to as the DASH diet (see below).

4.   Do not drink a lot of alcohol.

Diet affects high blood pressure. "DASH" stands for "dietary approaches to stop hypertension." Following the DASH diet and reducing the amount of sodium in your diet will help lower your blood pressure. If the pressure is presently normal, this diet will also help prevent high blood pressure, but its benefits extend to everyone, for it is low in saturated and trans fat, cholesterol, and total fat. It is rich in fruits, vegetables, and low-fat dairy foods. The DASH diet also includes whole-grain products, fish, poultry, and nuts. It encourages fewer servings of red meat, sweets, and sugar-containing beverages. It is rich in magnesium, potassium, and calcium, as well as protein and fiber.

To begin, the DASH diet requires no special foods and has no hard-to-follow recipes. Start by seeing how DASH compares with your current eating habits.

The DASH eating plan illustrated below is based on a diet of 2,000 calories a day. Your physician or a dietitian can help you determine how many calories a day you need. Most adults—depending on extraneous factors such as physical activity—need somewhere between 1600 and 2800 calories a day. Serving sizes for different foods vary from 1/2 cup to 1.25 cups. Check product nutrition labels for serving sizes and the number of calories per serving.

Make changes gradually. Here are some suggestions that might help:

1.	If you now eat 1 or 2 servings of vegetables a day, add a serving at lunch and another at dinner.

2.	Puree vegetables and add them into soups, stews, and sauces.

3.   If you have not been eating fruit regularly, or have only juice at breakfast, add a serving to your meals, or have it as a snack.

4.   Drink milk or water with lunch or dinner instead of soda, sugar-sweetened tea, or alcohol. Choose low-fat (1%) or fat-free (nonfat) dairy products so that you are eating fewer calories and less saturated and trans fat, total fat, and cholesterol.

5.   Read food labels on margarines and salad dressings to choose products lowest in fat and sodium.

6.   If you now eat large portions of meat, slowly cut back—by a half or a third at each meal. Limit meat to 6 ounces a day (two 3-ounce servings). Three to 4 ounces is about the size of a deck of cards.

7.   Have 2 or more meatless meals each week. Increase servings of vegetables, rice, pasta, and beans in all meals. Try casseroles, pasta, and stir-fry dishes, which have less meat and more vegetables, grains, and beans.

8.   Use fruits canned in their own juice. Fresh fruits require little or no preparation. Dried fruits are a good choice to carry with you or to have ready in the car.

9.   Try these snacks ideas: unsalted pretzels or nuts mixed with raisins, graham crackers, low-fat and fat-free yogurt or frozen yogurt, popcorn with no salt or butter added and raw vegetables.

10.   Choose whole-grain foods to get more nutrients, including minerals and fiber. For example, choose whole-wheat bread and whole-grain cereals. Although whole grains are a healthy choice, large

portions can lead to weight gain. A portion of grain is 1/2 to 1 cup. A cup of food is about the same size as your fist.

Use fresh, frozen, or no-salt-added canned vegetables.

This diet will allow you to limit your sodium intake to no more than 2300 milligrams per day.

Although the DASH eating plan is not designed for weight loss, it contains many lower-calorie foods, such as fruits and vegetables. You can make it even lower in calories by replacing high-calorie foods with more fruits and vegetables and eating smaller portions.

For more information, see the Guide to Lowering your Blood Pressure with DASH at:

www.nhlbi.nih.gov/health/public/heart/hbp/dash/dashbrief.pdf.

CHAPTER 17

Red Meat: Should You Curtail it?

Most of us are aware that red meat—when consumed in excess—is not a very healthy choice. But what constitutes an excess of this food, and how bad is it? So, let's take a closer look at these issues:

First, red meat may shorten your life! In 2012 scientists at the Harvard School of Public Health[25] evaluated results from more than 120,000 subjects in two studies and found that, after a period of 28 years, those who ate the most red meat (two or more servings per day) had a 30% higher risk of dying than those who ate only about 1/2 serving or less per day. They concluded that 8% of deaths in women and almost 10% in men could be prevented if people consumed less than half-a-serving of red meat per day. In their study, a single serving was roughly 3 oz. of cooked steak, hamburger, or pork chop, but only 1 oz of sausage, ham, or other processed meat, and 1/2 oz. of bacon. These results fell in line with earlier studies involving half-a-million people. From this I would conclude that you don't need to stop eating such meat entirely, but curtailing your intake to about once a week can eliminate most of the risk.

Second, red meat is not "heart or brain healthy." This means that the arteriosclerotic process resulting from consumption of this meat can lead to heart attacks and strokes, both resulting from closure of arteries supplying blood to the heart and brain. So even if you survive, you may impair the function of your heart or brain, and with it, your lifestyle could go out the window. The reason: Red meat is a major source of saturated fat in the average diet. This latter fat raises bad (LDL) cholesterol levels and contributes to hardening of the arteries (arteriosclerosis). But other compounds in this meat may contribute to these bad effects. These latter substances include salt, iron from blood, and also potentially harmful compounds that are created when meats are cooked at high temperatures. Another possible culprit in meat is carnitine, a substance that may, on its own, enhance arteriosclerosis by promoting bacterial growth in the bowel that produces excessive TMAO (trimethylamine-N-exide). This latter substance is capable of producing accelerated heart disease in animals, and higher levels are found in individuals suffering from overt heart disease. These early observations are speculative and require further study for definite conclusions.

Another threat red meat poses is a greater risk of developing type 2 diabetes, a condition further enhancing the risks of arteriosclerosis and other bad outcomes. Several studies have linked processed red meats to an elevated rate of this disorder, and this may also extend to unprocessed red meats as well. One example: Harvard researchers tracked more than 200,000 people for up to 28 years and found that the risk of diabetes increased by 32% for every two ounces of processed meat—and by 12% for every three ounces of unprocessed meat eaten per day. Numerous possible explanations have been advanced explain this relationship, but the meaning is clear for each person's eating habits.

Finally, there is a relationship between red meat and cancer. The American Cancer Society has weighed in on this issue with the following statement: "Limit consumption of processed meat and red meat. To reduce your cancer risk, eat no more than 18 oz. per week of red meats such as beef, pork and lamb, and avoid processed meat such as ham, bacon, salami, hot dogs, and sausage." After careful analysis, they found that the risk of colon and rectal cancer rises by about 20% for every serving red or processed meat consumed daily, with additional suggestive evidence that the risk may extend to other cancers such as pancreas, prostate, esophagus, or breast. How red meat could produce cancers is unknown, but there are two possible pathways:

1.   N-nitroso compounds—capable of producing cancers in experimental animals—are created by the nitrites used to color and preserve processed meats like bacon, sausage, and lunch meats. But even unprocessed red meat seems to increase levels of these compounds, possibly through the effect of iron attached to the blood contained in red meat (as opposed to white meat).

2.   When meats are cooked to well done at high temperatures, heterocyclic amines and polycyclic aromatic hydrocarbons are formed, and these compounds are carcinogenic, at least in animals. This latter danger can be reduced by cooking to less well done at lower temperatures, a measure that applies to all types of meat—red or white.

Finally, excessive consumption of red meat is environmentally unfriendly. About two-thirds of corn and soybean production in the U.S.A. goes for animal feed rather than for humans. Since it requires about 5-8 lbs. of feed to produce one lb. of beef or pork, this inefficiency results in excessive use of water and fossil fuels which in turn jeopardizes our environment at a time when the world can ill-afford this burden. Moreover, methane, a potent greenhouse gas, is produced by cattle and has 23 times the heat-trapping capacity of carbon dioxide. Adding further to this burden, in order to accommodate increasing farmland to feed animals, forests must be cleared, again causing us to lose a valuable means to clear carbon dioxide from our atmosphere.

So I can simply conclude that those cattle appearing incessantly on TV are passing along the correct advice—"Eat Mor Chikin"! (and Fish, too!).

CHAPTER 18

Red Wine and Cardiovascular Disease: "The French Paradox"

Moderate red wine consumption has long been thought to play a possible role in reducing the risk of heart disease. For instance, the French seem to suffer a relatively low rate of such disease despite diets rich in "risky" components such as animal fats (foie gras, red meat, etc.) Since the French drink copious volumes of red wine along with these diets, their low heart disease rate—called the French paradox—has been the cause of speculation that red wine might contain components that are protective against this disorder. The consumption of alcohol, however, in any form—approximately one or two ounces daily—has been believed to lower levels of this risk. But this latter relationship has been questioned by a recent review that suggested that selection bias and/or genetic factors might be responsible for reaching questionable conclusions[26]. Thus at present we are unable to determine whether alcohol *per se* could be the underlying protective ingredient in red wine. Moreover, we don't really know that consuming a comparable amount of non-alcoholic grape juice might be just as protective as an equal quantity of wine.

We may be getting closer to an answer to this paradox, because reservatrol, a component in the skin of red grapes has recently been shown to reduce markers in the blood stream that constitute danger signs for heart disease[27]. This lends more support for the hypothesis that red wine might indeed be more potent than just the alcohol it contains as a guardian against cardiovascular disease.

Reservatrol is present not only in red grapes but also in peanuts (especially sprouted), peanut butter, mulberries, cocoa powder, dark chocolate, blueberries, cranberries, and others. Commercially purified reservatrol can also be taken by tablet. Even if beneficial, however, we really don't know how much reservatrol daily might be needed to achieve such an effect. If we take the figures supplied by the recent research study noted above, 8 milligrams (mg) given daily as a supplement might be the right answer. To place this in perspective, red wine and grape juice contain about 0.2 to 5.8 mg per bottle (1 liter), and peanuts and cocoa powder contain about one half these amounts on a weight to weight basis.

So how should the average individual respond to this kind of information? Since definitive answers are not yet available, my suggestions are as follows:

If you already enjoy one or two glasses of red wine daily, no change is necessary. Perhaps adding occasional peanuts or dark chocolate would be helpful, provided calories from this source don't contribute to weight gain.

If you are a teetotaler, consider adding occasional red grape or cranberry juice to your daily diet, and, of course, peanuts or dark chocolate might be considered.

Given the lack of definite proof, I believe it's too early to recommend taking commercially prepared reservatrol, especially since the natural foods noted above may have additional features beyond resveratrol that may be protective in themselves.

CHAPTER 19

Arsenic in Food: What Are The Concerns?

Arsenic is present in the environment as a naturally occurring substance, or it may result from human contamination. It is present in water, air, soil, and foods. In foods, arsenic may be present in both organic and inorganic forms, the latter being the most toxic. The FDA has been monitoring the levels of arsenic in foods for decades, and in 2011, increased its testing. Tests included more than 1,300 samples, and with regard to rice, they found that among all types of white rice, the briefly boiled version tended to have the highest levels of inorganic arsenic, with an average of 114 parts per billion (ppb). Instant rice had the lowest, averaging 59 ppb. Medium-grain rice from California tended to have lower levels of inorganic arsenic than rice originating from other parts of the U.S. Also white basmati rice from California, India, and Pakistan contain an average of about half the amounts of most others. Although inorganic arsenic is a known carcinogen, there are no federal limits for it in juice, rice, or most other foods. Moreover, many arsenic-containing rice products are marketed to children and infants as "health foods," and children are far more susceptible to the dangerous effects of arsenic exposure. Research suggests that high levels of arsenic exposure during childhood are capable of harming a child's developing brain, producing neurobehavioral problems as well as cancer and lung disease later in life. This means parents must be careful to avoid serving their children food with significant levels of arsenic. This is especially true for rice beverages that are used as a milk replacement, which means that children under the age of 5 should not receive any rice drinks as part of a daily diet.

Recently, Consumer Reports released their analysis of arsenic levels in rice products, and the results added more reason for concern. Popular rice products including white rice, brown rice, organic rice baby cereal, and rice breakfast cereals, were all found to contain arsenic. They concluded; "In virtually every product tested, we found measurable amounts of total arsenic in its two forms. We found significant levels of inorganic arsenic, which is a carcinogen, in almost every product category, along with organic arsenic, which is less toxic but still of concern." The study not only found a significant amount of arsenic in many rice products on the market, but also that arsenic levels in the blood directly increase with greater rice consumption. Several products tested had more arsenic in each serving than the 5 parts per billion (ppb) limit for adults set by the EPA as safe.

Consumer reports concluded that it's not necessary to completely eliminate rice from the diet. In light of current evidence, the EPA's 5 ppb per day limit on arsenic is probably what we should shoot for. Many of the white rice products tested had fairly low levels of arsenic, and in the context of a few servings a week for an adult, it's probably not an issue. As for very young children and infants, serving them rice products in general should be avoided. Pregnant women should be cautious about their rice intake, and minimize their exposure to arsenic to protect their developing fetus; finding another safe starch to replace rice during pregnancy would be wise.

So if you choose to purchase white rice, buy a brand made in California like Lundberg. Their California White Basmati Rice has only 1.3 to 1.6 ppb arsenic per serving (1/4 cup uncooked), well below the safe limit. In addition, rinsing the rice before cooking and boiling it in a high water-to-rice ratio can help reduce the arsenic content significantly.

Brown rice, on the other hand, has significantly more arsenic than white rice and should be avoided or consumed rarely. Some of the brown rice brands tested contained at least 50% more than the safe limit per serving, and a few even had nearly double the safe limit. Note that some of the worst offenders for arsenic content are made from brown rice: processed rice products like brown rice syrup, brown rice pasta, rice cakes, and brown rice crisps. These processed products are commonly consumed by those following a "healthy" whole grain rich or gluten-free diet, but they clearly pose a significant risk of arsenic overexposure, especially if a person eats more than one serving per day. Obviously, brown rice is not a food that should be a dietary staple, or even eaten on a regular basis.

Aside from having a higher arsenic content, it's harder to digest. Despite a higher nutrient content of brown rice compared to white rice, the anti-nutrients present in brown rice reduce the bioavailability of many vitamins and minerals present. Moreover, brown rice also reduces dietary protein and fat digestibility compared to white rice. In short, brown rice is not a health food for a variety of reasons, and a higher arsenic content is simply another reason to avoid eating it. Nevertheless, brown basmati rice contains about 1/3 less arsenic than other brown rice groups, providing at least one less toxic choice from this group.

Some scientific evidence suggests that the risks of arsenic can be even greater than previously suspected. Recently, researchers in the United Kingdom and India published a study providing the first evidence that frequently eating rice can alter the basic structure of cells. The study measured damage to chromosomes in cells obtained from the urine of more than 400 adult study participants in an area of India with low arsenic in drinking water. Those who ate about 2½ to 3 cups of cooked rice per day containing more than 200 ppb of total arsenic possessed more genetically damaged cells—potentially carcinogenic—within than those eating rice with less arsenic. The study noted that more than 10 percent of the rice in China, Pakistan, and Bangladesh is estimated to have arsenic concentrations exceeding 200 ppb, while in the U.S., more than 50 percent of the rice is estimated to contain arsenic at those elevated levels. More research is needed to see whether the study's results would apply to Americans, who eat less rice and generally have better nutrition.

Extending observations to other food sources, The FDA found elevated levels of arsenic in beer after testing 65 samples, all of which the agency says included some form of rice as an ingredient. The results showed that 10 of them contained inorganic arsenic levels that ranged from 15 ppb to 26 ppb, significantly more than the federal drinking-water limit of 10 ppb for total arsenic. Based on its full data, the FDA is presently conducting a risk assessment as the next step in a process to help manage possible risks associated with the consumption of rice and rice products.

What You can do about Rice

Diversify your food consumption to include grains other than rice, and when consuming the latter, avoid brown rice in favor of the white variety, preferably produced in California. And when you do cook rice, rinse it first, and use a ratio of at least 6 cups of water to 1 cup of rice (draining the excess water afterward). For those who are trying to avoid gluten (usually a mistake, as noted in chapter 39), switching to rice as an alternative is a poor choice.

Other Food Sources of Arsenic

Certain juices can also be a source of arsenic. The FDA in July 2013 proposed an "action level" of 10 parts per billion for inorganic arsenic in apple juice, stating that the 10 ppb guidance to industry "will help keep out of the food supply even the occasional lot of apple juice" containing arsenic above that level. But is this enough? Not according to researchers at Consumers Union, who urged the agency to set a lower level in order to create an incentive for the marketplace to reduce levels of inorganic arsenic in apple juice and thereby reduce risk even further—not simply maintain the status quo.

But the fact that most of the apple-juice samples the FDA tested already had inorganic arsenic levels below 10 ppb is one reason Consumer Reports' safety experts concluded that the agency's proposed guidance doesn't sufficiently protect public health. In written comments submitted to the FDA, they urged the agency to set a tougher level, recommending a limit of 3 ppb of total arsenic for apple juice, but certainly no higher than 4.4 ppb. They pointed out that, in calculating the risks of arsenic exposure from apple juice, the FDA appears to have significantly underestimated how much juice children drink. A survey of parents conducted in 2011 found that more than 25 percent of children under age 6 consumed more than 8 ounces of apple juice, which was the highest daily consumption estimate used by the FDA, and 12 percent drank 16 ounces or more.

But, unfortunately, apple juice is not the only culprit. Consumer's Union also urged the FDA to set action levels for other juices, such as pear and grape, where tests have found inorganic arsenic levels much higher than 10 ppb.

What You can do about Juice

Limit children's consumption of apple and grape juice. Children up to age 6 should have no more than 4 to 6 ounces a day. Moderation should also apply to adults, but at least large quantities should be avoided until more research data become available.

☙CHAPTER 20❧

What to do About A Cold

The common cold is caused by a viral infection in the upper airways, sinuses, throat, and nose, although most apparent in the latter area. Uncommonly there may also be a mild fever. Despite the discomfort from the sneezing, sore throat, cough, and runny nose, happily it gets better on its own without requiring any special treatment, usually within a week—but sometimes a bit longer. At present there is no cure for this common illness. So, while waiting for it to disappear, what can we do to ease the symptoms without making things worse?

First, since they have no effect on the culprit viruses, contrary to the common misconception, antibiotics should not be employed. Using them will neither shorten the cold's duration nor prevent its spread to others. Moreover, the more we take antibiotics, the greater chance of producing resistant bacteria that could create mischief to others at a later time. Although delayed complications such as pneumonia are occasionally encountered in elderly individuals, fear of complications is not a good enough reason to prescribe antibiotics for the common cold[28]. A better approach would be to consult a physician if the cold seems to persist for over a week, causes a moist cough, or produces a fever for more than one or two days.

What about echinacea, an herbal product that supposedly treats the common cold? Although there are only a limited number of controlled trials, there is no convincing evidence it is effective. The herb is probably safe, for prior studies show rates of side effects to be similar in echinacea and placebo groups. Thus with or without it, the cold will resolve within 1 to 2 weeks anyway. The same can be said for vitamin C, which has been extensively studied and offers no significant benefit.

Although there are no total cures, the element zinc has been known for many years to have an inhibitory effect on cold viruses in the laboratory. But now there seems to be some substance surrounding this issue: According to an analysis of three large trials[29], zinc acetate lozenges are an effective way to alleviate and shorten symptoms. Overall, the study showed high dose zinc acetate lozenges shorten the duration of colds by 42%, concluding that the lozenges shortened the duration of nasal discharge by 34 per cent, nasal congestion by 37 per cent and scratchy throat by 33 per cent, and cough by 46 per cent. Unexpectedly, the duration of muscle ache was reduced by 54 per cent. Adverse effects of zinc were minor in the three studies. Therefore, the authors concluded that "zinc acetate lozenges releasing zinc ions at doses of about 80 mg/day may be a useful treatment for the common cold, started within 24 hours, for a time period of less than two weeks." Lower doses of zinc may not be as effective.

Unfortunately, zinc lozenges on the market either have too low a dose of zinc or contain ingredients that tightly bind to zinc ions, such as citric acid. Therefore, when searching for suitable products, one should obtain the acetate form, check the amounts of zinc in each lozenge, and prepare to use them repeatedly throughout the day in order for the total daily dose to reach 80 mg

Given the absence of any definitive cures, what can we do to relieve symptoms during the illness? First, take plenty of liquids, especially water, to combat dehydration that may result from the cold, especially in children. Although I am a fan of chicken soup, which can help to combat dehydration and help relieve subjective symptoms, there is little evidence that real benefit will accrue.

Another often overlooked simple method is the use of salt water gargle—if you make a solution consisting of ¼ teaspoon of salt dissolved in 8 ounces of warm water and gargle, your sore throat symptoms may be temporarily relieved, probably resulting from salt water's ability to draw excess fluid from inflamed tissue. Applying saltwater to the nasal passages, done with nasal drops, may be useful for loosening thick mucus, making it easier to expel, especially for young babies. Nasal saline drops may be a useful alternative to salt solutions for gargling, a futile endeavor for babies and very young children.

Another old trick is the use of steam inhalation, which usually helps alleviate symptoms of upper respiratory congestion. You can half fill a pan with water and bring it to the boil. Place the pan on a sturdy table; make sure there is a towel or heat-resistant mat under it. Then sit with your head over the pan and cover yourself with a towel. Mechanical humidifiers, either with cold are warm steam, are also effective and easier to use.

Getting plenty of rest will not only help alleviate some of the symptoms, and make you feel less miserable, it may also reduce the duration of your cold. One should get plenty of rest for as long as symptoms persist, at least until abatement of the general sense of fatigue and malaise that often accompanies the cold. Remaining at rest is also important to prevent the spread of infection. As a rule of thumb, stay away from work or school while you do not feel well. When you can't avoid proximity to others, cover your mouth with a tissue when you cough or sneeze, and throw it away into a trash can immediately, and wash your hands with warm water and soap.

What else can we do to relieve the symptoms? First, antihistamines have been a time-honored method to relieve the nasal congestion and promote easier breathing (chapter 32). Sedating (first generation) antihistamines may alleviate some cold symptoms, such as the watery eyes, runny nose, coughs and sneezes, but the newer agents, such as Allegra[R], Zyrtec[R] and Claritin[R] are less sedating and can be more useful.

Decongestants are medications that shrink the swollen membranes in the nose, allowing for easier breathing. There are oral or nasal decongestants, I prefer the nasal form, oxymetazoline (Afrin[R]) because each application lasts for several hours and tends to produce less "rebound" nasal congestion upon withdrawal. Nevertheless, persistent use for more than about five days might produce excessive nasal blockage. Patients with high blood pressure should use decongestants with caution, best accomplished under a doctor's supervision.

Cough medicines, available in numerous forms, are generally not effective and, therefore, their use should be discouraged.

Although a high fever may not be desirable, a slight fever is not such a bad thing—it helps the body fight off infections more rapidly. When your body temperature rises, viruses (and bacteria) find it harder to reproduce, and this also seems to ramp up the body's defense mechanisms. With the exception of the very young, physicians no longer recommend trying to bring a slight fever down.

Painkillers (analgesics) may be helpful. The standard analgesics such as aspirin, acetaminophen (Tylenol^R), or ibuprofen (Advil^R), used for many years, produce relief of general aches. Aspirin should only be taken by adults, not children, especially very young ones.

So, the bottom line is simple: Hang in there; the cold will go away by itself. Just don't make matters worse by over treating with useless remedies that include antibiotics.

CHAPTER 21

Dietary Supplements: Some Good, Some Useless, and Some Dangerous

During the past 25 years dietary supplements have rocketed in popularity in the U.S.A., reaching over $25 billion yearly in sales. Contributing to a misguided air of authenticity, they are offered in drugstores, supermarkets, and health-food stores. But what do we actually know about these products in terms of both safety and efficacy? According to a large survey conducted in 2013, 55% of respondents thought the government required supplement makers to include warnings about potential dangers and side effects on their products. They don't, meaning that safety issues are often ignored.

So let's run down a list of highly popular supplements, and the pros and cons for each:

Multivitamins: Many people believe they can promote general health and ward off serious conditions such as cardiovascular diseases and cancer. But the facts don't support these contentions. Clinical trials repeatedly fail to show benefit of multivitamin supplements to healthy people. But even worse, they can, under certain circumstances, be risky: Both vitamin A and calcium can be dangerous if taken in excess, especially when added to a normal diet. Adult males and females should not ingest a daily total of over 3,000 mg. of vitamin A. Total daily calcium intake should not exceed 2,500 mg. Vitamin D intake should not exceed 2,000 IU. So check to see how much you are getting in your regular diet and avoid supplements that cause the totals to exceed these levels.

Vitamin E: Originally touted to prevent cardiovascular disease, later studies have totally debunked this premise. More recently, supplements of vitamin E were suggested in the hope of preventing prostate cancer, but actual study pointed in the opposite direction: This vitamin actually increased prostate-cancer risk in men age 50 and older.

B Vitamins: Often thought to promote healthy metabolism and energy, the evidence refutes this contention in most circumstances. A normal diet contains an excess of B1 (thiamine), B2 (riboflavin), B3 (niacin), B6 (Pyridoxine), B12 (cobalamin), and B9 (folic acid). Unless your diet is deficient (see below), supplementation is a waste of money. Vegetarians, and people (especially the elderly) having difficulty with absorbing B12, may benefit from supplementation of this vitamin. Moreover, women who are or may become pregnant should consider supplementation with folic acid, 0.8 mg daily. The oral form of supplemental folic acid is usually absorbed better than that found naturally in food. One caveat, however, is that high doses of folic acid can mask B12 deficiency that can lead to serious physical problems.

Vitamin K: Believed to promote healthy blood clotting and protein synthesis and prevent cancer. The reality: Leafy greens and other vegetables provide more than enough to satisfy the body's need for this vitamin. Moreover, the normal bacteria that inhabit the bowel synthesize vitamin K and can make up any possible shortfall. There is no evidence that supplemental doses can prevent cancer. But there is a downside risk: Too much vitamin K can make the anticoagulant (blood thinning) drug warfarin (Coumadin[R]) less effective, a serious potential danger.

Fish Oil: This supplement is widely used with the intent to prevent and/or treat cardiovascular diseases. Although the evidence indicates that two or more servings of fish weekly is capable to reducing heart attacks and strokes, linking fish oil supplements to these diseases is less clear. Some evidence suggests that they may help, but the better choice is in the dietary consumption of the fish itself.

Calcium: An important mineral constituent of the body, calcium is often taken with the intent of building healthy bone, thus preventing osteoporosis and fractures. But the evidence does not support such claims. Even with supplemental consumption of over 1,000 milligrams daily, calcium has not been shown to prevent fractures in either premenopausal or postmenopausal women. Among the possible risks of high calcium intake, some studies suggest that it may increase the risk of heart disease.

Vitamin C: For many years high doses of this vitamin have been used for preventing and treating colds, heart disease, and cancer. Despite numerous studies, however, the actual evidence fails on all these counts. Although generally safe, a possible risk of high doses of supplemental vitamin C can lead to unhealthy buildup of iron in body tissues and organs, posing a risk to the occasional individual suffering from iron storage disease (hemochromatosis).

Vitamin D: This vitamin is important in bone and muscle health, nervous and immune system function, cell growth and reproduction, and moderating inflammation. Although controversial, its administration is alleged to ameliorate certain types of heart disease, hypertension (high blood pressure), diabetes, and possibly multiple sclerosis. Some research suggests it may prevent colon cancer, and—although controversial—other cancers as well. It's also associated with a reduced rate of depression in older people, and greater immunity against some infections. So far, however, few controlled prospective trials have investigated the potential benefits of vitamin D supplementation in preventing any of these problems.

Normally we obtain vitamin D through sun exposure and dietary intake. It is manufactured by the body, but the process requires exposure to ultraviolet light. Given the widespread use of sunscreen, however, to prevent skin cancer, up to 36 % of Americans are low on this vitamin. Food sources for this vitamin are limited, although some products such as milk are fortified. Natural sources include fatty fish such as catfish, salmon, mackerel, sardines and tuna; eggs; beef liver; and cod liver oil. Your doctor can perform a blood test to determine whether you are deficient of this vitamin. If you are found to be deficient, instead of risking sun exposure, dietary modification and/or supplemental vitamin D should be considered.

The latest US recommendations for the minimum daily requirement of vitamin D, or cholecalciferol—vitamin D3, the preferred form—are 600 IU (international units) for those under 70, and 800 IU for those older. These quantities appear to retard bone loss. Persons infrequently exposed to the sun, especially the elderly, and postmenopausal women may need 800–1000 IU daily. From a review of available information, I conclude that people who get at least 700 IU of vitamin D daily have denser bones, have better muscle strength, and are likely to suffer fewer falls and fractures than those who don't. The only caution is to avoid exceeding the government's safe daily upper limit of 2,000 IU.

Glucosamine/Chondroitin: This supplement is widely used in the effort to help repair cartilage and relieve suffering from degenerative joint disease (osteoarthritis). After many conflicting studies, however, a recent, more definitive large study showed that glucosamine was unable to relieve knee pain or cartilage loss in people with osteoarthritis. Although generally safe, this product would pose some risk to some people with shellfish allergies.

Some Supplements Definitely to Avoid

Unless there is compelling evidence of efficacy—which is seldom the case—supplements should generally be avoided. Three especially egregious products linked to serious dangers are the following:

1.   Kava, which is taken to relieve stress and anxiety, is capable of producing serious liver disease.

2.   Yohimbe (yohimbine hydrochroride), used to treat erectile dysfunction, is risky because the impure ingredient present in over-the counter preparations, can cause unpredictable effects on blood pressure, rapid heart rate, and other problems.

3.   Aconite, touted to relieve inflammation and joint pain, can cause nausea, vomiting, low blood pressure, respiratory system paralysis, heart-rhythm disorders, and even death.

Is Anything Worth Taking?

In general, normal diets contain more than enough to preclude the need for supplementation. If one has a demonstrated deficiency of any, then, upon the advice of a physician, supplementation may be justified. As noted above, in the case of vitamin B12, folic acid, and Vitamin D, supplementation can be useful.

CHAPTER 22

Artificial Sweeteners—Any Worth?

Because of the widespread availability and use of artificial, non-caloric, sweeteners we must examine their impact—if any—on health. This is especially important because, according to a recent survey, 71% of adults in the U.S consume 10% or more of their daily caloric intake from added sugars, and many of them, in the attempt to correct this problem, have turned in a big way to artificial sweeteners.

At present there are six such sweeteners on the market, all cleared as being safe by the FDA. The following discussion centers on the three most prevalent, which are aspartame, saccharin, and sucralose.

First, let's look in more detail about each of these substances:

Aspartame (Equal' , Nutrasweet') is a combination of 2 amino acids, aspartic acid and phenylalanine. It is about 220 times sweeter than sugar and leaves little aftertaste when consumed. One rare exception to its excellent safety record is that those who have phenylketonuria (PKU) cannot eat aspartame. This is because their bodies cannot metabolize, phenylalanine, one of its amino acids. Fortunately PKU is a rare, genetically inherited condition that is routinely screened for in early infancy, and this regularly allows for those individuals to avoid such substances in their diets. Otherwise, aspartame is one of the most researched sugar substitutes available in the United States, with more than 200 studies establishing its safety, and no adverse health consequences have been identified. Although there has been a lot of misinformation about aspartame since it came onto the market in 1981, studies have concluded that it specifically does not cause headaches, seizures, Alzheimer's disease, Parkinson's disease, lupus, or multiple sclerosis.

Saccharin (Sweet N Low) is the oldest sugar substitute, first discovered in 1879. It is 200 to 700 times sweeter than sugar, depending on how it is used. Saccharin leaves an aftertaste some people can detect. Earlier, safety was of some concern, and it used to carry a warning label indicating that it was known to cause cancer in laboratory animals. After extensive research on the safety of saccharin, however, the United States government passed a bill in 2000 confirming its safety and removed the warning label from food and drinks made with saccharin.

Sucralose (Splenda) is another no-calorie sugar substitute that tastes like sugar but is 600 times sweeter. It leaves no aftertaste when consumed. It was approved for use in the United States in 1998, and also has been subjected to many studies on its safety, all of which have indicated that it is safe for people to consume in customary amounts used for sweetening.

How Effective Are These Products? Since we have recognized their excellent safety record, another important question centers on whether they are helpful:

Although substitution of artificial sweeteners in food and drinks offers promise of better weight control, I note that leading medical organizations have weighed in on this issue.[30]

According to the joint scientific statement from the American Heart Association and American Diabetes Association. "At this time, there are insufficient data to determine conclusively whether the use of such sweeteners to displace caloric sweeteners in beverages and foods reduces added sugars or carbohydrate intake, or benefits appetite, energy balance, body weight, or cardiometabolic risk factors."

As suggested, research results are mixed about this issue, because some studies show that individuals consuming artificial sweeteners often compensate by consuming more high caloric foods in response to the non-caloric sweeteners, thus nullifying any efforts at weight control. Although this is a complicated issue, from personal experience I have found virtually nothing to suggest that those individuals consuming such products actually do lose weight. One counter argument, however, is to say that these same individuals—had they consumed sugary beverages—would have actually gained weight, but, unfortunately, they probably would have done so either way. Accumulating evidence[31] demonstrates that frequent consumers of sugar substitutes are actually at increased risk of excessive weight gain. This may result because consuming sweet-tasting but non-caloric or reduced-calorie food and beverages interferes with learned responses that normally constrain sugar and energy consumption. As a result of this interference, frequent consumption of high-intensity sweeteners may have the contrary effect of inducing metabolic or brain responses that actually induce the individual to eat more calories. Some experimental studies in animals have also supported this contention.

Not only has research failed to confirm the idea that artificial sweeteners are beneficial in reducing overall caloric sugar intake, there are some preliminary data suggesting that they may be actually harmful, increasing one's propensity to develop cardiovascular disease, i.e., the same malady that we wish to prevent. These newer data show an association between daily consumption of dietary beverages and cardiovascular disease (CVD) outcomes (including mortality) in postmenopausal women. The findings were based on an analysis of dietary beverage intake and cardiovascular risk factors in 59,614 women who did not have cardiovascular disease at the time they enrolled in the study. Results were reported in March, 2014, at a large national medical meeting. At an average follow-up of 8.7 years, they found that women who drank at least two diet drinks on a daily basis had a higher risk of cardiovascular disease (CVD) events compared to the zero-to-three drinks per month group. A newer study[32] conducted over a 9 year period in individuals over 65 years old also showed that, after adjustment for multiple potential confounders, waist circumference increases of 2.04 cm for non-users of diet drinks, 4.67 cm for occasional users, and 8.06 cm for daily users. Unfortunately, this added weight accumulated in the belly regions, increasing further the risk of diabetes and cardiovascular disease.

Almost all researchers caution that this type of research, although showing clear links between artificial sugar intake and CVD, does not conclusively establish a causal role for such beverages, because other, heretofore unrecognized factors may cast such a conclusion in doubt. Nevertheless, at this time it falls on the makers of diet drinks to show that they are free of harm.

Regardless of the eventual resolution of this issue, however, simply substituting all sweetened/caloric beverages with simple unadulterated water is the best—and cheapest—solution to this problem. If you cannot tolerate plain old water, seltzer or unsweetened tea may be an acceptable alternative. In the absence of conclusive data, children and pregnant women are advised to avoid any of these products.

CHAPTER 23

Why Junk Food is "Double Trouble"

Michael Moss's recent book entitled "Salt Sugar Fat: How the Food Giants Hooked Us," has provided us with more good reasons why junk food is dangerous to our health, but most importantly, how it contributes mightily toward the obesity epidemic that has been "growing" all about us. Having moved beyond one form of dangerous products, the tobacco companies have purchased much of the processed food industry, and, similar to their cigarette promotions, they are now passing on their sneaky tactics to entice people into consuming their newly acquired unhealthy food products.

In the book, Moss quotes James Behnke, the former Pillsbury executive. "We're hooked on inexpensive food, just like we're hooked on cheap energy. Unfortunately, much of this revolves around price sensitivity and the growing disparity between the haves and have-nots. It costs more money to eat fresher, healthier. And so there is a huge economic issue involved in the obesity problem. It falls most heavily on those who have the fewest resources and probably the least understanding of what they are doing."

So below are a few tips to help you avoid succumbing to the companies' various methods of subterfuge:

Foods are Branded to Look "Natural."

Apparent grill marks on hamburgers are often faked. They are put there by factories to possess a natural appearance. Ironically, in order to possess these marks, the food requires more processing than ever. Rather than switch to ingredients that are healthier and less processed, food engineers at companies with notoriously processed products such as Kraft, Wendy's, McDonald's, and Dominos—among others—are responding to concerns about processing with an unhealthy and deceiving façade of healthy looking foods. Kraft Foods engineers spent two years manufacturing a Carving Board line process that would create uneven turkey slabs, and Wendy's intentionally created curvier "natural squares" out of perfectly square beef chunks so they would appear less processed. And the list goes on and on.

Marketing to Children Under the Guise of Charity

Unfortunately, childhood obesity has more than doubled in the last 30 years. More than a third of children and adolescents are now overweight or obese, and the numbers are increasing. One example of sneaky marketing is supplied by McDonalds, who may take an entire elementary class on a lunchtime "field trip" to hear from Ronald the clown about Ronald House Charities, while, at the same time, to partake in their unwholesome foods. This suggests that by eating such products, you are doing a "good deed" for society. In addition, they often employ social media, branded "advergaming" websites, which include videogames that are supposedly educational, but in reality are actually marketing ploys.

Manufacturing Addiction

Despite knowledge to the contrary, many people continue to crave junk food, primarily because the companies that produce it have scientifically created "feel-good foods," containing just the right combination sugar, fat and salt that

94

our brains adore. This moves us toward a "bliss point," which is the optimum combination that the brain likes best. The companies' so-called "pillar ingredients" consist of salt, sugar, and fat, combined in just the right way as to keep you hooked. The processing includes "mouth feel," i.e., the crunchy sensation that consumers most crave. They also employ the so-called "flavor-burst," by altering and shaping salt crystals in order to induce a flavor that can basically assault the taste buds into submission. Finally and perhaps most importantly, is the concept of "vanishing caloric density," which underlies all junk-food science. This is the process by which the food melts in your mouth so quickly that the brain is tricked into believing that it is consuming fewer calories than are actually present. The packaged-food scientists want you to avoid the sensation of satiety that tells a person to stop eating when it is overwhelmed by flavors. This tends to foster extra eating unassociated with the hunger sensation. This promotes both heftier sales together with matching body weights.

How to Reduce the Amount of Processed Foods You Eat

Processed food is literally everywhere and generally unhealthy. But here are a few simple tips provided by Michael Moss that will help you eat both healthier and less:

1.   *Seek True Satisfaction:* Enjoy genuine flavors, rather than fat, sugar, and salt added to mask the metallic taste of chemical additives.

2.   *Read Labels Wisely:* You can find food with "real" ingredients in a supermarket by avoiding those showing a long list of ingredients, which is usually a sure sign that it's processed in an unhealthy way.

3.   *Relish What's On Your Plate*: Devote time solely to enjoying the pleasures of eating.

4.　　*Wean Yourself Off Excess Salt, Fat, and Sugar*: You can also cook with smaller amounts of these ingredients by using natural substitutes like strong spices.

5.　　*Give Your Palate Time to Change:* You'll gradually lose your taste for excessively sweet and salty foods.

6.　　*Go For High-Quality Foods:* Look for products that contain the least amount of processed ingredients.

7.　　*Do Not Skip Meals:* Try eating three meals a day at fairly regular times, but try to minimize or avoid eating when you are not hungry. Regular eating at mealtimes will leave much less of an urge to snack or seek out a vending machine. If you must snack, try eating any variety of nuts, especially unsalted varieties.

8.　　*Last But Not Least:* Eat lots of fruits and vegetables!

C✍CHAPTER 24✌

Smoke Inhalation: How Bad Is It?

Cigarette smoking is a serious problem, accounting for at least 440,000 deaths annually in the United States. As compared to nonsmokers, smokers suffer an average reduction of longevity by approximately twelve to fourteen years. But smoke inhalation causes deaths that include much more than the usual suspects of lung cancer and heart disease (Table 1). It now accounts for at least 21 diseases that include approximately 15 types of cancer and a variety of at least 22 other diseases.[33,34] And to make matters even worse for smokers, recent data has linked this exposure to kidney failure, intestinal damage from reduced circulation, and numerous types of infections. This means that the total number of deaths in the U.S.A. due to smoking was likely underestimated, and now likely exceeds 500,000 yearly. But there is some good news for the smokers: In general the risk for each of these maladies declines progressively with the number of years after quitting.

Diseases Caused by Smoking

Cancers

1. Oral
2. Larynx

3. Esophagus

4. Lung

5. Leukemia

6. Stomach

7. Liver

8. Pancreas

9. Kidney

10. Cervix

11. Bladder

12. Colon

13. Breast

14. Prostate gland

15. Unknown source

Other Diseases

1. Stroke

2. Blindness

3. Cataracts

4. Macular degeneration

5. Pneumonia

6. Maternal smoking: Congenital defects

7. Periodontitis

8. Aortic aneurysms

9. Coronary heart disease

10. Hypertension (High blood pressure)

11. Tuberculosis

12. Asthma

13. Diabetes

14. Reduced fertility (women)

15. Ectopic pregnancy

16. Hip fractures

17. Erectile dysfunction (ED)

18. Rheumatoid arthritis

19. General infections

20. Kidney failure

21 Intestinal blood flow restriction

21. Peripheral vascular disease

Present estimates also extend this mortality to non-smokers regularly exposed to ambient smoke (secondary smoke) by as many as 40,000-45,000 annually. In recognition of this latter problem, many municipalities nationwide have passed ordinances prohibiting smoking in public places. As a result, the rate of hospitalizations for numerous ailments attributable to smoke inhalation has fallen accordingly. These conditions include heart attacks, strokes, and lung cancer.

Our state, Indiana, has responded favorably to this information: Beginning July 1, 2012, nearly all public places, including restaurants and other workplaces, are now smoke free. This change comes as the result of Indiana's first ever statewide smoke free air law, designed to protect Hoosiers from the harmful effects of exposure to secondhand smoke, which contains 200 known poisons and 43 cancer-causing agents. Nevertheless, smoking continues to be permitted in the following places: bars and taverns, tobacco retail shops, cigar and hookah bars, licensed gaming and horse track facilities, and, under certain circumstances, membership clubs.

But how realistic is it to allow these exceptions noted above? Are we performing a disservice to the non-smoking employees and patrons of these latter facilities by permitting their continued exposure to such toxic exposure? The risk in these environments was recently disclosed in a recent study, published in an American Heart Association journal[35], as summarized: Drawing information from the years 2000 through 2012, the researchers noted that on July 1, 2006, the state of Colorado implemented a state law that made all work and public places, restaurants, and bars smoke free, but casinos were exempted. This was followed by an impressive (22.8%) drop in ambulance calls to all these aforementioned facilities, but no change in calls to casinos. On January 1, 2008, however, the law was extended to include casinos, and as a result, these latter places then enjoyed a comparable reduction (19.1%) in such emergency calls, while, at the same time, similar reduced calls to the other public places held steady at already established reduced rates.

This study could not detail the exact causes of the emergency calls, but the conclusions appear inescapable: Although we have long known that environmental smoke is unhealthy in the long run, its effects also become apparent in a surprisingly short time. Indiana is not alone in allowing casinos and the like the right to smoky exposure, for as recently as April 2013, only 19 states plus Puerto Rico had laws making all state regulated gambling sites smoke free. Moreover, most tribal casinos are also not smoke free. This means that workers and patrons of such facilities are being subjected to unnecessary risks.

The dangers of toxic air pollution extend to auto emissions. Living near major roads appears to increase the risk of heart disease and sudden cardiac death, at least in women.

A team from Brigham and Women's Hospital and Harvard University evaluated data from 107,130 women who were part of the Nurses' Health Study (1982 - 2012); 532 of the participants suffered sudden cardiac death, and, in total, 1,159 died from coronary heart diseases[36].

After adjusting for other influencing factors, living close to a major road (within 50 meters, about 150 feet) compared to living at least half a kilometer (about one-third mile) away, increased the risk by 38 per cent. For each 100 meters closer, the likelihood of sudden cardiac death was six per cent higher.

On a population level, therefore, the risk factor for sudden cardiac death when living close to heavy traffic was comparable to other known influencing factors such as smoking, diet or obesity, said main author Jaime E. Hart. Living close to traffic also raises the risk for the development of lung cancer, as shown in another study[37].

Conclusion:

Those who have an option to avoid indoor tobacco smoke exposure are advised to do so, but for those who do not have such a choice, public regulation is required. We owe it to those involuntarily trapped in these places such as casino employees, to press for more legislative action as soon as possible. Living near areas of heavy traffic and other polluting sources is much more difficult to avoid. Perhaps this may provide more impetus to curbing consumption of fossil fuels.

CHAPTER 25

Electronic Cigarettes (E-Cigarettes): Good, Bad, or Indifferent?

An electronic cigarette (or e-cigarette), electronic vaping device, personal vaporizer (PV), or electronic nicotine delivery system (ENDS) is an electronic inhaler meant to simulate and substitute for tobacco smoking. It generally employs a heating element that vaporizes a liquid solution. Some release nicotine, while some merely release flavored vapor. Although they are often designed to mimic traditional cigarettes in their appearance, more devices are not trying to imitate them. To this date the benefits and risks of these products are uncertain, but they are likely safer than smoking tobacco. Laws vary widely concerning their use and sale, and are the subject of pending and ongoing debates.

E-cigarettes are the latest fad sweeping this country. Their sales increased from 50,000 in 2008 to 3.5 million in 2012. As of 2011, in the United States, one in five adults who smoke has tried electronic cigarettes. Hon Lik, a Chinese pharmacist, is widely credited with the invention of the first generation electronic cigarette. In 2003, he came up with the idea of using an ultrasound-emitting element to vaporize a pressurized jet of liquid containing nicotine diluted in a propylene glycol solution. This design produces a smoke-like vapor that can be inhaled, and provides a vehicle for nicotine delivery into the bloodstream via the lungs. The device was first introduced to the Chinese domestic market in May 2004 as an aid for smoking cessation and replacement. The company that Hon Lik worked for started exporting its products in 2005–2006. Several e-cigarette models marketed by tobacco companies were launched or were set to launch in 2013, including the Vuse, MarkTen, and Vype. Blu, a prominent e-cigarette producer, was also acquired by Lorillard Inc., a tobacco industry leader, in 2012.

Smokers have access to these products and, unless bad effects surface, they are unlikely to be banned in the near future. Since non-smoking children occasionally try them, they should be prevented from access to these products without parental consent.

So are these "cigarettes" effective in aiding smokers in their attempts to quit? To answer this, a clinical trial[38] in 2013 evaluated the comparative efficacy of 16 mg. nicotine e-cigarettes, nicotine patches (21-mg patch, one daily), or placebo e-cigarettes (no nicotine). All were adult smokers and wanted to stop smoking. This study lasted for 13 weeks and smoking abstinence was assessed after 6 months. Although not dramatic, the e-cigarettes did show a modest rate (7.3%) of abstinence versus a 5.8% rate with the patches and 4.1% rate with the placebo. Other studies have shown similar—or even less impressive—results. Complicating this issue further, other studies frequently reveal that most people who use e-cigarettes are so-called "dual users," meaning that they use e-cigarettes in addition to paper-and-tar cigarettes, pointing toward no progress toward quitting the latter.

But are e-cigarettes safe? Unfortunately we have no long-term safety data on the impact of repeated inhalation of propylene glycol or vegetable glycerin on lung tissue. Some short-term data suggest that they may cause airway (bronchial) irritation, but to what extent and how that compares to standard cigarettes are unknowns. Even more worrisome, however, they have also been found to contain potentially harmful irritants, genotoxins, and carcinogens. Preliminary studies in animals suggest that exposure to this vapor may even interfere with the body's ability to resist various infections, especially involving the lungs. Marked inter-device and inter-manufacturer variability of e-cigarettes, which use various chemicals and aerosolization techniques that result in variable nicotine and contaminant delivery, makes it hard to draw conclusions about the safety or efficacy of the whole device class[39].

Currently, e-cigarette manufacturers are devoting attention toward manufacturing and marketing rather than creating reliable scientific data about these products. Theoretically, if these products contain only nicotine and no other known carcinogens they should at least reduce the risk of cancer.

So where do we stand regarding whether we should recommend use of these products? I conclude with points below:

1.   At present, e-cigarettes are not clearly superior to Food and Drug Administration-approved medications for smoking cessation.

2.   They are not yet FDA approved for treatment.

3.   Short-term safety data suggest they may cause lung irritation.

4.   Long-term safety data do not exist. Until recommending these products, we need more data.

5.   Although the jury is still out, they may be worth a try for someone who is desperately trying to quit smoking and has failed other means.

Thus at present we are largely in uncharted waters.

CHAPTER 26

A Few Tips About Pain-Killers

The nonsteroidal anti–inflammatory drugs (NSAIDs) are used to treat mild and moderate pain due to many non-serious conditions, including osteoarthritis (degenerative arthritis of aging), headaches (including migraines), menstrual periods and muscle soreness. With 70 million prescriptions each year in the U.S., NSAIDs are one of the most commonly used types of medications.

Let's focus here on osteoarthritis (degenerate joint disease of aging), which affects about 27 million Americans, according to the National Institute of Arthritis and Musculoskeletal and Skin Diseases. Although it occurs in younger people, it's seen most commonly in adults age 65 and older.

A good way to treat osteoarthritis, if medication is needed, is with an NSAID. These drugs block the production of substances in the body called prostaglandins, which play a role in pain, inflammation, fever, and muscle cramps and aches. At low doses, NSAIDs work essentially as pain relievers. At higher doses, though, they not only relieve pain but can actually reduce the body's inflammatory response and may minimize tissue damage.

Most oral forms of NSAIDs are now available as less expensive generic forms. And three are available in lower-dose formulations as nonprescription over–the–counter drugs: acetylated salicylates (Aspirin[R], Bufferin[R], and generic), ibuprofen (Advil[R], Motrin[R], and generic), and naproxen (Aleve[R] and generic). Although their costs vary from about $4 to more than $300 a month, sticking to those noted above will save lots of money, but first discuss with your doctor about the medicine and dose that is right for you, along with possible risks.

All NSAIDs should be used with caution, because they can cause serious side effects, including stomach ulcers, gastrointestinal bleeding, heart attack, stroke, and liver and kidney damage. Most NSAIDs (except for low–dose aspirin) may not be appropriate for people at risk of heart disease or stroke. In any event don't take them for long periods of time without consulting a physician.

A newer type of NSAD, in a class termed "COX-2 Inhibitors", as exemplified by celecoxib (Celebrex[R] may reduce gastrointestinal irritation, but in addition to posing a risk for cardiovascular events, is not superior to the older NSAIDs in relieving pain (See Chapter 59).

My two favorite choices are noted below (both available over-the-counter)

1.   Ibuprofen – (Advil, Motrin and generic)

2.   Naproxen – (Aleve and generic)

These two medicines are inexpensive and are as effective and safe as other NSAIDs when used appropriately. Following are some of the points to consider:

1.   If you have had a peptic ulcer or intestinal bleeding, or are at high risk of either, avoid using NSAIDs. The risk of bleeding from NSAID use

increases with age. Even if you're not having such problems, try to avoid taking any of this class of drugs on an empty stomach.

2.   If you have heart disease or are at risk of heart attack or stroke, talk with your physician about the potential risks of taking any NSAID regularly for long periods, especially at high dosage levels. Of all the members of this category, naproxen appears to be nearly free of these cardiovascular risks.

3.   Take the lowest dose of an NSAID that brings relief and do not take any longer than necessary.

4.   If you have kidney disease or high blood pressure, talk with your physician about the risks of taking NSAIDs for long periods of time.

5.   NSAIDs can interact with other medicines to cause serious side effects. If your doctor prescribes an NSAID, tell him or her about any other medicines or dietary supplements you are taking.

CHAPTER 27

Heartburn: Some Important Facts and Suggestions

Acid reflux, a frequent cause of chest pain, commonly felt as "heartburn," afflicts as many as 40% of our entire population. It is caused by inadequate closure of the muscular door that guards against upward flow from the stomach into the esophagus, a tube that objects to acid being applied to its lining. But reflux can do more than cause the pain we call heartburn: It can cause postnasal drip, hoarseness, difficulty swallowing, chronic throat soreness and clearing, coughing, and even wheezing and shortness of breath that mimics asthma. Complicating this issue further, reflux can occur in the absence of telltale chest pain or indigestion, occasionally surfacing only in the form of the aforementioned respiratory symptoms.

Annual sales of standard anti-acid medications, used to combat this problem, now exceed $13 billion. These medications include a myriad of products that range from the non-prescription agents such as Maalox[R] and Tums[R], to the various blockers of stomach acid production such as Zantac[R] or Nexium[R], and many others. What's even more troubling is that reflux can increase the risk of developing esophageal cancer later in life, which has increased by about 500% since the 1970s. The commonly used antacids not only fail to protect against the long-term risk of cancer, but, paradoxically, for uncertain reasons, may actually raise the risk to an even higher level. The current American lifestyle appears to have accounted for the widespread increase in the reflux problem: This includes the combination of obesity with poor dietary habits that include sugar, soft drinks, fat, and processed foods. But also a major culprit is the delay of dinnertime to later evening hours, often after 7:00 p.m., frequently including a gargantuan meal consisting of fatty foods, chocolate, and wine, all of which contribute to delayed emptying of the stomach together with increased acid production.

So what can we do about this common problem? In addition to the standard oral antacid preparations, a major change that often succeeds is the reduction of the size of your evening meal, combined with not eating after 7:00 p.m.—or at least not eating for three or more hours before bedtime, and avoidance of the bad dietary constituents noted above. Gravitational forces created by lying flat in bed also promote acid reflux, and therefore, raising the head of the bed during sleep can provide much relief. By raising the head, however, I do not refer to simply using more pillows, but the entire upper body must be elevated through the use of a wedge under the upper mattress or placing blocks under the legs of the bed at the head end to elevate the upper portion by at least six to twelve inches.

If you have any of the symptoms noted above, or wish to achieve a healthier lifestyle, you might wish to try these simple measures—preferably after consulting with your physician.

CHAPTER 28

Can We Prevent Premature Aging of The Skin with Sunscreen?

We have long been aware that excessive exposure to the sun's ultraviolet rays is associated with an increased rate of skin cancer as well as exaggerated aging of skin. But can we conclude that, by using common sunscreens, we can avoid these undesirable consequences? In the case of at least one type of skin cancer (*squamous cell cancer*), the evidence is compelling that sunscreen can prevent this disorder.

But, until now, even though logic dictates that we can retard aging of the skin with sunscreen, rigorous scientific studies—i.e. randomized, controlled investigations—have not been applied to answer this question.

Now, recently appearing in a prominent medical journal[40] are the results of just such a trial, and the answer is clear: The study included 903 mostly Caucasian adults younger than 55 years at the outset. They were randomly assigned into four separate groups. One group applied a broad-spectrum sunscreen daily, while the remaining groups were instructed to apply the sunscreen at their own discretion. The study was continued for 4 1/2 years with careful study of the skin surfaces by skilled examiners who were unaware of which subjects were receiving which treatments. Included in this study was an evaluation of beta-carotene (source of vitamin A), an agent alleged to have "antioxidant" properties postulated to prevent skin aging.

Results: The daily sunscreen group displayed no detectable increase in skin aging after 4 1/2 years, which amounted to 24% less than those who applied sunscreen only by discretion. Interestingly, the beta-carotene failed to retard this aging process.

These authors used a sunscreen labeled "sun protection factor 15+," but qualified this with the following statement: "Whether our results would have differed with a sunscreen with a higher sun-protection factor or one with greater absorption in the ultraviolet spectrum is debatable, because the overriding factor in achieving adequate skin protection is application of a liberal quantity of sunscreen; the sun-protection factor or precise shape of the sunscreen-absorption spectrum is far less important."

Conclusion:

Although this study leaves some questions open, certain conclusions seem inescapable: We can indeed retard aging changes of the skin in Caucasians with sunscreen, but daily widespread and liberal applications are required, at least on days that one is exposed to any sunshine whatsoever. But will it produce similar effects in older individuals whose skin is already seriously weathered? And can we extend this information to include darker skinned races? These latter points will require further study.

With regard to beta-carotene, this study adds further evidence against one more of the touted benefits from "anti-oxidants." As I have noted before, the entire concept that oxidation is harmful within the body is unproven at best, and flawed at worst.

Finally, you might ask which sunscreen products are the most cost-effective. Although Consumer Reports covers this in detail, two products are especially worth considering:

1.   Equate (Walmart) is a lotion that carries a protection factor of 50.

2.   Up & Up (Target) is a spray that has a similar protection number.

CHAPTER 29

Sleep Nice or Pay The Price!

Most people, having busy schedules, often resort to cutting down on their hours of sleep. But even minimal sleep loss takes a toll on your mood, energy, and ability to handle stress. The quality of your sleep directly affects the quality of your waking life, including your mental sharpness, productivity, emotional balance, creativity, physical vitality, and even your weight. No other activity delivers so many benefits with so little effort.

Sleep isn't exactly a time when your body and brain shut off. While you rest, your brain stays busy, overseeing biological maintenance that keeps your body running in top condition, preparing you for the day ahead. Without enough hours of restorative sleep, you won't be able to work, learn, create, and communicate at a level even close to your true potential. As you start getting the sleep you need, your energy and efficiency will go up. In fact, you're likely to find that you actually get more done during the day than when you were skimping on shuteye. You may not be noticeably sleepy during the day, but losing even one hour of sleep can affect your ability to think properly and respond quickly. It also compromises your cardiovascular health, energy balance, and ability to fight infections. Loss of sleep during the week leads to accumulated "sleep debt" that can only be partially repaid by extra sleeping during weekends.

Both the quantity and quality of sleep are important. Some people sleep eight or nine hours a night but don't feel well rested when they wake up because the quality of their sleep is poor. The best way to figure out if you're meeting your sleep needs is to evaluate how you feel as you go about your day. If you're logging enough sleep hours, you'll feel energetic and alert all day long, from the moment you wake up until your regular bedtime. Extra sleep nightly can relieve problems of excessive daytime fatigue. Some people can avoid a sleep deficit by taking short daytime naps. Older adults also often have trouble sleeping this long at night; daytime naps can help fill in the gap.

How Much Sleep Do You Need?

Although there is some genetic variation, most adults require 7 to 9 hours of sleep per 24-hour period to function optimally.

Of course age plays an important role in sleep requirements. According to the National Sleep Foundation, newborns (up to three months) a daily sleep duration of 14 to 17 hours is recommended, for infants (four to eleven months) twelve to 15 hours, for toddlers (one to two years) eleven to 14 hours. At pre-school age (three to five years) the experts recommend ten to 13 hours of sleep, for school children (six to 13 years) nine to eleven hours. For teenagers, the ideal sleep duration is recommended at eight to ten hours, for adults (18 to 64) seven to nine hours. Older adults (above the age of 65) are advised to sleep seven to eight hours.

Most adults can find their optimal sleep time by setting aside several days (perhaps during a vacation) to allow sleeping as long as possible. After this time is determined, it's best to allot that amount of time in one's daily schedule for sleep.

Sleep Deprivation Can Even Add to Your Waistline

Most of us who are short on sleep crave sugary foods that may impart a quick energy boost. There's a good reason for that. Sleep deprivation has a direct link to overeating and weight gain. There are two hormones in your body that regulate normal feelings of hunger and fullness. Ghrelin stimulates appetite, while leptin sends signals to the brain when you are full. However, when don't get the sleep you need, your ghrelin levels go up, stimulating your appetite so you want more food than normal, and your leptin levels go down, meaning you don't feel satisfied and want to keep eating. So, the more sleep you lose, the more food your body will crave.

Health Dangers of Inadequate Sleep

Previous studies have shown that inadequate amounts of sleep are associated with a higher long-term mortality risk. A recent study has shed more light on this subject, at least when evaluating sleep duration in combination with other well-known factors that lower one's survival outlook.

In the National Institutes of Health-AARP Diet and Health Study (1995-1996), researchers examined associations among sleep duration and various causes of death. They studied cardiovascular disease and cancer mortality among 239,896 US men and women aged 51-72 years who were free of any of these diseases at the beginning of study. They evaluated the influence of moderate-to-vigorous regular physical activity, television viewing, and body weight on the interplay between sleep and mortality.

Compared with 7-8 hours of sleep per day, shorter sleep durations were associated with higher total mortality, especially due to cardiovascular diseases. Especially noteworthy was a higher cardiovascular mortality in those with lesser sleep among overweight and obese people, suggesting a special interaction between reduced sleep and overweight. People in the unhealthy categories of all four risk factors—sleep less than 7 hours/day, less than one hour of vigorous physical activity weekly, television viewing greater than 3 hours/day, and moderate to severe overweight—had an all-cause greater risk of dying approaching 50% greater than that of those lacking any of these factors. Although deaths in this group were most likely attributable to cardiovascular disease, they surprisingly also had higher than normal rates of cancer.

Although this study does not provide any single answers, it adds further support to the idea that adequate sleep is highly desirable, but it needs to be buttressed by the other lifestyle factors that we all recognize as conducive to better health.

A Few Tips for Better Sleep

For the reasons presented above, getting enough good-quality sleep is essential to staying healthy and aging well. Certain sleep problems—for example, sleep apnea—require medical treatment. As noted, lack of sleep can have serious consequences—a higher risk of, obesity, type 2 diabetes, heart disease, and other health conditions. It can also raise the risk of falling, particularly among older women, and, if you drive, it increases the likelihood of having a car accident. Insomnia might also leave you feeling anxious, depressed, or irritable. Paying attention, learning, or remembering can become difficult. So here are a few simple steps that can help you overcome insomnia:

Stick To a Consistent Sleep Schedule and Routine

Go to bed at the same time each night and wake up at the same time each morning. A set sleep routine will "train" you to fall asleep and wake up more easily.

Use the Bed Only For Sleep and Sex

No explanation necessary.

Cut Down on Caffeine

For some people, even a single cup of coffee in the morning means a sleepless night. Caffeine can also increase the need to urinate and interrupt sleep during the night.

Be Physically Active

Regular aerobic exercise like walking, running, or swimming provides three important sleep benefits: you fall asleep faster, attain a higher percentage of restorative deep sleep, and awaken less often during the night. But try not to exercise shortly (less than 3 hours) before retiring, for it temporarily raises your body's temperature and metabolic rate, factors that can transiently interfere with sleep.

Limit Daytime Naps

Prolonged napping can disrupt your natural sleep cycle and prevent you from feeling tired enough to fall asleep.

If You Use Tobacco in Any Form, Quit

Nicotine makes it harder to fall asleep, although this is the least of all its evils.

Use Alcohol Cautiously

Alcohol depresses the nervous system, so a nightcap may help some people fall asleep. But this effect disappears after a few hours and may lead to waking up throughout the night. Alcohol can also worsen snoring and other sleep breathing problems.

Improve Your Sleep Surroundings

Remove the television, telephone, and office equipment from the bedroom. This reinforces the idea that this room is meant for sleeping. An ideal environment is quiet, dark, and relatively cool, with a comfortable bed and minimal clutter. If you are accompanied by someone who snores loudly, use of earplugs or background steady noisemakers may be helpful, but moving to separate sleeping quarters may be required.

If You're Still Awake after About 20 Minutes in Bed

Get up and read awhile to relax. Otherwise, you'll set yourself up for tossing and turning.

Try to Avoid Sleeping Pills

If you do take a prescription sleep medicine, work with your doctor to use it effectively and for as short a time as possible. If you must take medicine, I prefer short-term generic zolpidem (Ambien), which is fairly effective and inexpensive. Another type of inexpensive medication is melatonin, a non-prescription substance normally produced in humans by the pineal gland, which is located in the center of the brain. Although not the sole regulator, it is involved in the sleep-wake cycle. Its production is inhibited by light and stimulated by darkness, which seems related to a mild ability to promote sleep.

Sleeping Pills are Especially Dangerous to The Elderly

Unfortunately, between 8 and 35 percent of the population over 65 consumes such pills, often on a regular basis. The so-called benzodiazepines are the most widely used for both insomnia and anxiety. The brand names include

Ativan, Ambien, Halcion, Klonopin, Lunesta, Sonata, Valium, and Xanax. (Some, like Ambien and Lunesta, actually belong to a class of sister drugs but have the same effects on the brain.) But they all present a problem—especially given older users' changing metabolisms and the likelihood that they're taking many other drugs. Such people taking sleeping pills are five times more likely to report poor concentration and memory, and twice as likely to have hip fractures and car accidents. They also experience more incontinence.

Despite these risks, however, many older people keep taking these drugs because they're psychologically addicted, believing they can't function without them. They may have unrealistic ideas about how much sleep older adults actually need—most 80-year-olds will do fine with six hours a night. It's normal for older people to wake up a couple of times a night, but they don't like it. The best countering strategy—after the risks above are explained—is to wean them off the pills over 12 to 20 weeks, allowing the blood levels to go down slowly. In the process, there may be a few nights of trouble sleeping, so they should just plan their activities accordingly. Eventually, the body will catch up.

C✦CHAPTER 30✦

Back Pain: A Common Problem Often Misunderstood and Over-Treated

lmost 80% of our entire population encounters at least one bout of lower back pain during their lifetime. More than 50% of Americans suffer from some type of low-grade chronic back pain. In approximately 90% of these cases, x-rays and other imaging studies of the back show no clear abnormalities to explain the discomfort. Such pains are probably caused by muscle strain and spasm that may be produced or aggravated by emotional tension. Patients over 40 often have minor degenerative changes of the spinal column in X-ray images, but these rarely produce symptoms. The central nervous system and brain may also enhance the sensation of pain, and this may be manifest by increased sensitivity to painful stimuli in other parts of the body[41].

Fortunately, serious spinal disorders are seldom the cause for back pain, which, in the case of recently acquired pain, usually resolves spontaneously within two weeks, regardless of what is done. The diagnosis is usually based on exclusion of specific physical abnormalities such as a herniated disc in the vertebral column. Therefore, in this setting, too many people receive premature high-tech expensive tests, powerful painkiller drugs, or even surgery.

Because the pain may be excruciating, most people seek medical help very early, are aggressively managed, and, as a result, waste money. Instead of helping, this approach may actually slow one's recovery. Low back pain is defined as acute when it persists for less than six weeks, sub-acute between six weeks and three months, and chronic when it lasts longer than three months. Certain findings, called red flags, point toward the likelihood that the pain may have a more serious underlying structural cause[42]: These include, among others, associated leg pain with or without numbness and weakness, feeling generally unwell, weight loss, and discomforts extending beyond the back. Other markers (yellow flags) point toward a strong likelihood that the pain will become chronic: These include obesity, depression, anxiety, frequent pains extending beyond the back, job dissatisfaction, and others[43].

Not surprisingly, many sufferers from back pain turn to chiropractors, and indeed many large surveys show that patients believe chiropractic works for them. Studies that compare patients' satisfaction with chiropractic versus conventional treatment in management of low back pain, show a preference for chiropractic treatment, which, ironically, has not been shown to be more effective than conventional physical therapy[44].

The results of a survey of over 14,000 subscribers conducted by *Consumer Reports* echo those of other studies; 58% of respondents reported that chiropractic treatments "helped a lot." They also noted that spinal manipulation can be helpful for lower-back pain in the short-term, but Consumers Union, the publisher of *Consumer Reports*, cautions that manipulations can aggravate structural problems, such as a herniated disk. For chronic back pain lasting more than 12 weeks, however, chiropractic did not appear to be better than general medical care, including physical therapy, exercises, and weight reduction. Chiropractic treatment carries one additional warning: Manipulations extending to the neck carry a slight but definite risk of damage to the spinal cord or proximal blood vessels, both of which can lead to serious—or even fatal—outcomes. Thus elderly patients, especially with preexisting disease of the vertebral column or blood vessels (arteriosclerosis), should be advised to avoid any manipulation of the neck.

So the following comments may help you understand and react to back pain in an appropriate way:

1. In the case of recent onset of pain—even if intense—do not rush to get tests such as X-rays or MRI scans. In most cases the pain will resolve spontaneously, and anything found in such testing will not help in recovery. Moreover, as mentioned, minor abnormalities found in these pictures only contribute to anxiety rather than resolution of pain. Moreover, in the case of X-rays, the radiation exposure produces a small but definite risk of developing cancer later in life.

2. Although recommended for years, try to avoid lying down for extended periods. Recent studies have shown that if limiting rest in bed to no longer than four days,, resuming normal activities results in less pain and earlier recovery. Activities should be low in impact such as stretching and walking, with light exercises that strengthen your abdomen, back and legs. Applying heat to the painful areas may be helpful.

3. Avoid the use of strong drugs such as opiates (OxyContin, Percocet, hydrocodone, etc). Use instead the so-called non-steroidal analgesics such as ibuprofren (Advil), naproxen (Anaprox), and

others. The opiate drugs are more apt to lead to more disability after several months and may even lead to addiction.

4. Some measures that also may be helpful include the following: Tighten your belt, which can help strengthen stomach muscles, a maneuver than can protect the back. Sit forward and straight in chairs, for that relieves strain of the back muscles. Try to sleep on your back or side, and when supine, place a pillow under your knees. Back massage, which can be done by a physical therapist, may help to relieve muscle spasm and the associated pain.

5. Avoid needless surgery: Back pain often stems from problems that cannot be helped by surgery, such as poor posture, minor arthritis, weak muscles, and others. Even when the pain is caused by conditions such as a herniated disk or spinal stenosis (narrowing of the spinal column), conservative treatment is often enough. Surgery might be considered if you have severe back and leg symptoms clearly linked to a herniated disk or spinal stenosis that hasn't improved with conservative treatment in three months. But even then, additional measures might first be tried such as local injections with anti-inflammatory agents or analgesics. In recent years, surgical treatment for chronic back pain (defined as that persisting for 3 months to a year) has fallen into disrepute[45]. This is because active nonsurgical management, consisting of rest, heat, massage, and analgesic medications, sometimes combined with psychological support (which may modify one's understanding of his or her pain and disability through mental restructuring

methods such as attention diversion, or by altering maladaptive thoughts, feelings, and beliefs) have been shown to provide just as much benefit as surgery for patients in whom there is no evidence of compression of spinal nerves. We medical practitioners often encounter patients who have undergone one or more surgical procedures without relief, and to me, that represents a real tragedy.

ᴄᴘCHAPTER 31ᴇᴏ

The Many Positive Benefits of Regular Exercise

Few people realize that the benefits of regular exercise extend far beyond just physical fitness and the resulting sense of well-being. What's really special is that, to be beneficial to the average adult, exercise need not be of Olympic proportions: By this we mean 30-60 minute sessions at least three times weekly that include almost any activities from brisk walking to strenuous aerobic workouts. The many benefits obtained stem from solid medical research. The ways that exercise helps us are almost too numerous to detail. Its effect is well known in preventing and treating heart disease and strokes, and in reducing and preventing elevated blood pressure levels.

At this point, however, one might ask whether there is a minimum level of exercise below which benefits are lost, and also whether one can be too old to gain from physical activity. Surprisingly, every small bit seems to count, with no age limit. In one large study[46], researchers analyzed exercise data from 1,170 people aged between 74 and 84. By recording and comparing sedentary periods with slow walking and moderate walking or equally intensive activities, they evaluated age, cholesterol levels, blood pressure, and other measures. From this they were able to assess participants' 10-year heart risk. They found that excessive sitting each day was associated with elevated risk, as opposed to progressive risk reductions with low to moderate activities. This information suggests that, even in the elderly, simply replacing sedentary existence with light activities of all types may confer important benefits that probably include decreased risk as well as better bodily function and mobility.

Mental Benefits from Exercise

A positive attitude is one of the best and immediate benefits of exercise: Not only do normal people feel more upbeat for extended periods of time, but many studies have shown that exercise is an effective way to combat serious depression. It is so effective for this purpose, it seems to equal or exceed the benefits obtained from those ubiquitous antidepressant medications constantly blaring on the TV commercials.

And all these benefits come at a cheap sticker price—a deal that's hard to beat! Other important ways that exercise is beneficial are explained below.

Exercise and Cancer

For the past 20 years, evidence has been accumulating that exercise can prevent some cancers, especially those involving the colon and breast. The list of potentially preventable cancer types has been growing, with evidence now suggesting that the prevention may also include cancers of the lung, esophagus, uterus, and prostate gland.

Regarding cancer in men, prostate cancer is one of the most prevalent forms, being diagnosed in approximately 223,000 men yearly, but fatalities are relatively low, at 29,000. This is followed by lung cancer (total 110,000, deaths 88,000) and colorectal cancers (total 72,700, deaths 27,000).

In women, a whopping 230,480 new cases of invasive breast cancer are being diagnosed yearly in the U.S., of which a total of 39,500 are expected to die from this disorder.

The National Cancer Institute[47] has provided an extensive review of this subject: In 2003, a paper in the journal *Medicine & Science in Sports & Exercise* reported that more than a hundred population (epidemiologic) studies on the role of physical activity and cancer prevention have been published. The authors noted that:

"The data are clear in showing that physically active men and women have about a 30-40 percent reduction in the risk of developing colon cancer, compared with inactive persons ... With regard to breast cancer, there is reasonably clear evidence that physically active women have about a 20-30 percent reduction in risk, compared with inactive women. It also appears that 30-60 min/day of moderate- to vigorous-intensity physical activity is needed to decrease the risk of breast cancer, and that there is likely a dose-response relation."

These studies were collected mainly by questionnaires about exercise regularity and subsequent development of cancers. Although this type of information is convincing, we now have even more conclusive results derived from careful assessment of physical fitness and development of cancer, at least in men, as noted below.

According to a 20-year, prospective study of more than 17,000 men at the Cooper Institute in Dallas, Texas[48], levels of measured cardio respiratory fitness appear to be as predictive of cancer risk and survival as they are of heart disease risk and survival.

Their data showed that the risks of lung and colorectal cancer were reduced 68% and 38%, respectively, in men with the highest level of fitness, compared with those who were the least fit.

Although fitness did not significantly reduce prostate cancer incidence, the risk of dying was significantly lower among men with prostate, lung, or colorectal cancer if they were more fit in middle age.

Although prior studies have shown that being physically active is protective against cancer, this study is unique because it looked at a very specific marker—cardio respiratory fitness as measured by maximal exercise tolerance testing. What was unexpected was that evidence of fitness not only predicts prevention of cancer but also even mortality after cancer has already been diagnosed.

Thus quantitative measurements of fitness might be compared with measuring your cholesterol, providing us with a very specific number to target. Merely asking someone about his/her physical activity may not provide that information.

The 17,049 men in the study underwent exercise testing with a treadmill or bicycle and risk factor assessment at an average age of 50 years as part of the long term study. Metabolic equivalents (METs) were used to record the men's fitness and to place them into five graded groups. Lung, colorectal, and prostate cancers were assessed.

Follow-up data were recorded over twenty years. Compared with men in the lowest fitness group, hazard ratios for developing lung and colorectal cancer men in the highest fitness group were 68% lower for lung cancer and 32% lower for colorectal cancer, even after researchers adjusted for such risk factors as smoking, body mass index, and age. In men who had already developed all these cancers, mortality also declined in the higher fitness groups.

These findings indicate that everyone can benefit from improving their fitness. The study did not evaluate whether a particular type of exercise contributed more consistently to cardiovascular fitness, but in general, activities performed at high intensity, regardless of type, seemed to be the best way to improve fitness and provide the most optimum results.

Additional research is needed to determine fitness and cancer risk in women, fitness and risk of all major site-specific cancers and the necessary change in fitness to prevent cancer.

In the meantime, plenty of exercise is fit for all!

Exercise and Alzheimer's Disease

Several studies have shown that regular exercise could prevent the occurrence of Alzheimer's disease (dementia). This was further supported by a large study[49] in which a preventive medicine clinic studied midlife fitness levels and the subsequent development of all-cause dementia in advanced age, and the findings were quite illuminating, especially because of the large numbers of persons studied and the length of follow-up: The project followed 19,458 community-dwelling, non-elderly adults who had a baseline fitness examination by means of a treadmill test. They eventually encountered 1659 cases of dementia covering literally thousands of person-years of follow-up (median time of follow-up, 25 years). After adjustment for several extraneous variables, those individuals showing the highest fitness levels demonstrated a much lower likelihood of developing dementia than the group with the lowest fitness levels, a difference that averaged a striking 36%.

These researchers concluded that higher midlife fitness levels were associated with a lower risk of developing any type of dementia later in life, regardless of its cause. Why the brain responds so favorably to exercise is uncertain, but at least one previous study[50] that used brain imaging showed that brain shrinkage, normally found in aging, could be retarded by regular exercise, a finding that raises intriguing possibilities.

Of course, studies of this type are always subject to limitations, but the researchers concluded; "all these gathering results should be taken seriously, especially since high levels of fitness confer so many other health benefits free of any significant long-term risks." Perhaps we might conclude that one is never too fit not only for body, but also for mind!

Exercise and Body Fat Distribution

It is well known the regular exercise reduces the percentage of fat carried by the body, especially important if it is distributed around the waist and abdomen. Such fatty deposits often lead to the development of dangerous tendencies such as diabetes and cardiovascular disease.

But to what age do these directives extend? Researchers from the University of Illinois have shown—as in the case of adults—that normal weight children should undertake regular physical exercise. Their study[51] divided 220 eight- and nine-year old children into two groups. The intervention group trained five times per week for 70 minutes over a nine-month period with moderate to vigorous physical activity. They measured before and after cardio respiratory fitness, fat content, abdominal fat content and its composition. The control group had no training targets.

After the nine months, no change of fitness in the control group was found. Compared to the intervention group, the children in the control group increased the body fat percentage and the abdominal fat structure. Thus, there was a marked difference between the two groups. "The initial weight did not play a role," said study author N.A. Khan, adding further that "The weight of healthy-weight children who don't exercise enough doesn't remain stable; normal-weight children who don't exercise gain an excess amount of weight for their age. When they become overweight, there is a tendency that the fat will be stored in the abdomen." That clearly goes in the wrong direction, warns the author, and advises parents to urge their children to exercise regularly.

Thus it appears that exercise is good for humans at every age, and it probably cannot begin too soon.

Exercise Increases Pain Tolerance

Finally, regular exercise may even alter how a person experiences pain, and this has been analyzed extensively[52]. For some time, scientists have known that strenuous exercise briefly and acutely dulls pain. As muscles begin to ache during a prolonged workout, the body typically releases natural opiates, called endorphins, and other substances that can slightly dampen discomfort. This effect usually begins during the workout and lingers for perhaps 20 or 30 minutes afterward.

But whether exercise alters the body's response to pain over the long term and, more pressing for most of us, whether such changes will develop if people engage in moderate, less draining workouts have been unclear.

So a more recent study[53] employed six weeks of exercising, using a program of moderate stationary bicycling protocol in volunteers for 30 minutes, three times a week, for six weeks. In the process, the volunteers became more fit, and these volunteers were compared to a control, non-exercising, group. As expected, the control group showed no changes in their responses to artificially induced pain. But those in the exercise group displayed a substantially greater ability to withstand pain. Although the pain began at similar threshold levels, their tolerance had risen. Those volunteers whose fitness had increased the most also showed the greatest increase in pain tolerance.

Results such as these suggest that those who exercise do not find the pain as threatening after exercise training, although discomfort is still experienced, an idea that fits with entrenched, anecdotal beliefs about the physical fortitude of athletes.

Pain tolerances were tested using people's arms and the exercisers trained primarily their legs, and this suggests that something occurring in the brain was probably responsible for the change in pain thresholds, a really intriguing idea.

The study's implications are considerable and indicate that the longer and more vigorously we stick with an exercise program, the less physical pain of any type we are apt to feel. The brain probably begins to accept that we are tougher than it had thought, and it allows us to continue longer, although the pain itself is still present.

This study also could be applicable to people struggling with chronic pain of all types, such as those suffering from "fibromyalgia," a poorly defined condition characterized by widespread muscular pains. Although anyone suffering from chronic pains of any cause should consult a doctor before starting to exercise, this type of experiment suggests that at least moderate amounts of exercise can change peoples' perception of their pain and help them to be able to better perform activities of daily living. When coupled with the other multiple health advantages of exercise, the implications should be obvious to all of us.

CHAPTER 32

Nasal Allergies: A Few Tips

Nasal allergies are common, afflicting almost everyone from time to time[54]. Although not usually a serious disorder, this type of allergy is a nuisance with symptoms of sneezing, nasal discharge and itching, and sometimes nasal obstruction and cough. The technical term for this condition is *allergic rhinitis,* meaning simply allergic nasal inflammation. Its common causes are seasonal pollens and molds, as well certain indoor allergens such as dust mites, pets, pests, and some molds. These nasal allergies usually begin during early infancy, arising first from indoor contacts, then later from outdoor pollens. This condition builds to peak prevalence from ages 10 to 30, and then usually gradually recedes thereafter.

Although this is a worldwide problem, nasal allergies seem to be increasing in western countries, now exceeding 40% in many areas of the U.S. and Europe. Although not life threatening, they contribute to missed time at work and school, sleep problems, and in children, limitation of outdoor fun. Adding to this outdoor restriction, children suffering from such allergies are more likely to have ear infections, tonsillitis, and asthma. Adding further to these woes, up to 40% of those with nasal allergies will at some time develop asthma. Moreover, those with nasal problems are more apt to develop conjunctivitis (eye inflammation) and even certain allergic skin eruptions (eczema).

Being more commonly found in relatives, heredity plays an important role is this disorder. Interestingly however, those children with older siblings or who grow up on a farm are less apt to develop nasal allergies, possibly as a result of multiple exposures to microbes that alter the immune system in some unknown way.

A nasal inflammatory reaction may persist after a single exposure to the offending agent, and may last for hours. Enhanced sensitivity to other contacts such as strong odors and other irritants may also persist for more extended periods and complicate the picture further. Thus the situation is more complex than simply an acute reaction to a single allergen.

How this Condition is Recognized

Recognition is usually simple, since the nasal symptoms regularly occur in response to a particular allergen and responds—at least in part—to an oral antihistamine. Proof can be further substantiated through blood or skin testing, but that is seldom necessary. Occasionally some individuals suffer from a form of "non-allergic" nasal symptoms, a form that may be a response to unknown allergens or irritants. Confusion can also occasionally arise when seasonal viruses account for similar symptoms.

What to Do

Depending upon the severity of the symptoms, a variety of options is available for management.

Treatment usually begins with an oral antihistamine, and most are obtainable without a prescription. The older ("first generation") members of this group are effective against the symptoms but produce more drowsiness, and for this reason, they are often less desirable. This group is represented by Benadryl (diphenhydramine), Chlor-Trimeton (chlorpheniramine), Vistaril (hydroxyzine), Phenergan (promethazine), and Tripohist (triprolidine). On occasion, however, their sedating effects can be an advantage, for they can promote sleep, relieve anxiety, and combat motion-sickness, and thus may be preferred when the situation requires any of these features.

The so-called "second generation" antihistamines are relatively free of sedation and thus better suited for purely combating the nasal allergy. Members of this group are Zyrtec (cetrizine), Claritin (loratadine), Allegra (fexofanadine), and Xyzal (levocetirizine). Although all are effective, personal preference may favor one of them, and possibly Allegra may be least sedating by a small margin.

Several of the antihistamines are available as nasal sprays by prescription, and they appear to be about as effective as their oral counterparts.

When the effect of the oral antihistamines is not complete, as is often the case, they can be combined with the oral decongestant Sudafed (pseudoephedrine). Combination preparations such as Actifed (pseudoephedrine with triprolidine as the antihistamine) were initially available, but in 2006, in response to legal issues, pseudoephedrine was declared a prescription item. Actifed's U.S. formula was changed to phenylephrine as the decongestant, chlorpheniramine maleate as the antihistamine. Nasal sprays containing the decongestant, Afrin (oxymetazoline) can be more effective for this purpose at least in the short term, but if used for longer than approximately 3 days, may produce a type of "rebound" nasal congestion unrelated to the allergy itself.

Cortisone type steroid (glucocorticoids) sprays can be given intranasally once daily, and provide at least moderate relief of seasonal nasal allergies, probably equal to the antihistamines. For instance, Nasacort (triamcinolone) is now available without a prescription. Although relief from these agents is obtained within one day, their peak effect may not be reached for several weeks. When combined with the antihistamines, they usually afford maximum relief.

Another group of medications, the so-called leukotriene-receptor antagonists, given by prescription, can also provide useful adjuncts for control of nasal symptoms. This latter category consists of Singulair (montelukast) and Accolate (zafirlukast). Although they are more commonly associated with control of asthma, they can provide modest relief of nasal allergy and can be added to the antihistamines, but probably add no relief beyond the combination of glucocorticoid sprays with antihistamines.

Immunotherapy

In general surveys, about one to two thirds of sufferers fail to achieve good relief from treatments noted above. The next step in treatment is with so-called "allergen immunotherapy," in which the patient receives the offending allergen in increasing concentrations until a maintenance dose is reached. This had always been done by injections under the skin, but more recently, rapidly dissolving tablets under the tongue have been approved for treatment of at least grass and ragweed allergy. Treatment then continues at the maintenance dose level, given once a month, for at least three years. This type of treatment seems to down-regulate the allergic response by mechanisms that are not well understood. The good news about this approach is that the beneficial effects often last for at least three years after the therapy is discontinued. Although serious allergic reactions may follow properly administered treatments, they are exceedingly rare, about one in one million.

Conclusion:

The comments above should help you move in the right direction in control of nasal allergy. Most instances can be managed on one's own, bolstered by the various non-prescription medications. Beginning with an antihistamine, this, in itself may suffice to control the symptoms, possibly with an added decongestant. If necessary, a nasal steroid spray can be added. Regardless of which direction one takes, always look for the most inexpensive, usually generic, agents to select as the preferred choices.

MYTHS

ᴄ✺CHAPTER 33✺ᴐ

Belief in Conspiracy Theories About Health

Apparently, nutty ideas, once widely disseminated, are often impossible to dispel. Over the past 50 years, numerous conspiracy theories have arisen about cancer, cell phones, spread of HIV infection, genetically modified foods, vaccines, water fluoridation, and alternative medical treatments. What remains unclear is whether the American public supports such conspiracy theories and whether they correlate with actual health behaviors.

A recent study[55] found that health-related conspiracy beliefs are indeed common. Researchers who studied the responses of 1351 U.S. adults to an online survey have concluded that conspiracy beliefs are widespread and are correlated with various health-related behaviors. For example, 37% believed that the FDA is intentionally suppressing natural cures for cancer because of drug company pressure; 20% thought that corporations were preventing public health officials from releasing data linking cell phones to cancer; 20% that doctors and the government still want to vaccinate children even though they know such vaccines to be dangerous; and 12% believed that fluoridation is really a secret way for chemical companies to dump dangerous waste products into the environment. Overall, 49% agreed with at least one medical conspiracy theory, and 18% agreed with three or more. The study also found that belief in conspiracies correlates with greater use of "alternative" medicine, i.e., treatments that lack scientific confirmation of efficacy, together with avoidance of scientifically supported medicine. The so-called "high" believers were more likely to buy farm-stand or "organic" foods and use herbal supplements and less likely to use sunscreen or get flu shots or annual checkups.

As I explain in many of the following chapters, anyone who believes and behaves according to any or all the above nonsensical information is doing so at one's own risk, possibly even placing his/her own very life—and that other family members—in jeopardy.

CHAPTER 34

Some Irrational Fears Never Die

A dangerous myth arose from a study published in 1999[56], describing a small group of twelve children who were supposedly normal until after they received a standard immunization (MMR) to prevent measles, mumps, and rubella (German measles). These children presumably developed autism in the aftermath, leading to the premature conclusion that immunization caused the mental problems. In contrast to generally accepted valid science, however, the numbers in this study were far too small to allow any real conclusions, and, therefore, carefully controlled studies would have been necessary to establish that the immunizations were responsible. Nevertheless, this report ignited a worldwide scare over vaccines in general and autism—and caused millions of parents to delay or decline potentially lifesaving immunizations for their children. Subsequently numerous independent studies were performed and failed to find any link between vaccines and autism. Moreover, procedural problems were uncovered involving the original publication that impugned the integrity of the original study, causing the author to be discredited and the journal editors to retract the entire study.

Unfortunately, vaccination rates in England and worldwide plummeted after the study was originally publicized. By the year 2012, nearly 40% of American parents also have declined or delayed a vaccine, according to the Center for Disease Control. Many parents now have a vague distrust of vaccines—with little to no memory of diseases that terrified their grandparents. Thus the myth continues and places many children at serious risk for development of easily preventable diseases that extend far beyond the diseases mentioned above. Vaccines are necessary because a massive amount of research has proven their effects in allowing millions of people to avoid disease and death. This dates back more than 200 years with the conquering of smallpox, to the present day, with similar advances in controlling polio, measles and many others.

We are now learning that contracting measles carries even more, heretofore unknown risks: Damage caused to a child's immune system by the measles virus can last for up to three years, leaving them highly susceptible to a host of other serious diseases. A new study, published in the journal Science, has shown that children, after suffering from measles, have impaired immunity to other, nastier diseases, raising their later odds for lethal outcomes. These findings suggest that measles vaccines have benefits that extend well beyond just protecting against measles itself.

Defying logic even to this day, a recent study of messages designed to reduce vaccine misrepresentations and increase vaccination rates has found that pro-vaccine messages do not always work as intended and sometimes have the opposite effect[57]. The study involved 1759 parents who have children in their household age 17 or younger. Parents were randomly assigned to receive 1 of 4 interventions: (a) information explaining the lack of evidence that MMR causes autism, (b) textual information about the dangers of the diseases prevented by vaccination, (c) images of children who have diseases prevented by vaccines, or (d) a dramatic narrative about an infant who almost died of measles. None of the interventions appeared to increase parental intent to vaccinate a future child. Refuting claims of an vaccine/autism link successfully reduced misperceptions that vaccines cause autism; nevertheless, those parents who had the least favorable vaccine attitudes continued to resist future plans to vaccinate. In addition, showing parents images of sick children increased expressed belief in a vaccine/autism link, and a dramatic narrative about an infant in danger increased self-reported belief in serious vaccine side effects.

Conclusion:

Current public health communications about vaccines may not be effective. For some parents, they may actually increase misperceptions or reduce vaccination intention. Attempts to increase concerns about communicable diseases or correct false claims about vaccines may be especially likely to be counterproductive. More study of pro-vaccine messaging is needed.

Individual counseling during which parents voice their fears may be more effective but can require considerable time. It might also be useful to try to decrease the spread of misinformation through mainstream media channels.

Unfortunately, people who believe vaccination is unnecessary are often responding to misleading scare tactics as promoted by pseudo-scientific groups such as the National Vaccine Information Center, that despite its official sounding name, has no creditability among the scientific world. For many years, this group has hosted anti-vaccine conferences to argue that vaccines can cause serious adverse effects. Unfortunately, this has provided a platform for a number of well-known charlatans that include Andrew Wakefield (responsible for the original misconception) and Mark Geier, who have lost their medical practice licenses. I will withhold other names that are also notorious. Most counter-arguments consist of anecdotes or individual "testimonials" of dire consequences following a vaccination, similar to the original discredited example of autism described above.

I conclude with a quote from Paul A. Offit, MD, Chief of the Division of Infectious Diseases and the Director of the Vaccine Education Center at the Children's Hospital of Philadelphia: "I think the media have got to be far more responsible about covering this issue. If you look at the way it was covered fifteen years ago, it was always a false mantra of balance, which is tell two sides of the story when only one side is supported by the science...I think the media are much more responsible about this now because the outbreaks are so egregious that you can't help but feel the choice not to get a vaccine was a bad one."

Unfortunately, the problem persists, and thus this is my best effort to help in correcting the myth and calming the fears.

CHAPTER 35

Energy Drinks: What's All the Hype About?

They're all over the place, brazenly claiming to keep you revved up, energized, and alert. But controversy is now raging over these products, for several deaths have reportedly followed their use. So we need to explore the facts about these drinks.

First, how do they accomplish this energy infusion? I can answer with a single word—caffeine! We all know it is the active ingredient in coffee. An 8 ounce cup of coffee contains about 100 milligrams of caffeine. By contrast, a 16-ounce Starbucks Grande contains about 330 milligrams. That's why most people drink coffee in the morning: It's a helpful "waker-upper" to get them started and ready to attack the day with a head of steam. But now we encounter other products that claim to accomplish the same (or better?) feat. Despite containing a variety of vitamins and extraneous substances, these products actually exert their influence with that self-same ingredient, i.e., caffeine. So in order to clarify this issue, Consumers Union recently tested a whole slew of these drinks—27 in all—and came up with some interesting results: Caffeine levels per serving ranged from about 6 milligrams to 242 milligrams—and some containers included more than one serving. The highest caffeine content was in 5-hour *Energy*

Extra Strength. Although all brands don't list actual content, 5 of the 16 products that list a specific amount of caffeine— Arizona Energy, Clif Shot Turbo Energy Gel, Nestlé Jamba, Sambazon Organic Amazon Energy, and Venom Energy— contained more than 20 percent above their labeled amount on average in the samples they tested. On the other hand, one of three samples of Archer Farms Energy Drink Juice had caffeine about 70 percent below the labeled amount. For the other tested drinks that list caffeine levels, the actual numbers were within 20 percent of that claimed, which were thought to be an acceptable range for meeting caffeine claims. Eleven of the 27 drinks tested didn't specify the amount of caffeine. Were they harboring some dark secret? Their blends might have been proprietary, for some include amino acids, carbohydrates, or guarana (a botanical caffeine source). A response from the Monster Beverage Corporation provided another reason for the absence of listing: "because there is no legal or commercial business requirement to do so, and also because our products are completely safe, and the actual numbers are not meaningful to most consumers." Nevertheless, labels on two tested Monster drinks warn against use by children, pregnant or nursing women, and people sensitive to caffeine. The Monster drinks and eight others also recommend a daily limit.

Various scientific groups have for years urged the Food and Drug Administration to require disclosure of caffeine levels, but the agency says it lacks the authority to do so. So what do we conclude? According to Consumers Union, "although caffeine can make you feel more alert, boost your mental and physical performance, and even elevate your mood, it can also make you jittery, keep you from sleeping, cause rapid pulse or abnormal heart rhythms, and raise blood pressure. Safe limits of caffeine consumption are still being studied, but data suggest that most healthy adults can safely consume up to 400 milligrams per day; pregnant women, up to 200 milligrams; and children, up to 45 to 85 milligrams depending on weight." My advice: Stick to coffee, considering the caffeine limits cited above. Forget the "energy drinks." They are a waste of money.

CHAPTER 36

The Fortified Food Myth

Today the fastest growing category in the food industry is so-called "functional food"— fortified food that's supposed to reduce your risk of disease or boost your chances of optimal health, according to the marketers. There is some support for adding certain elements to standard foods, such as calcium, fiber, omega-3 fatty acids, and certain vitamins. Overall, such altered foods account for $20 to $30 billion in annual sales, says Price Waterhouse Coopers. And sales of fortified foods are predicted to grow at an annual rate of 8.5 to 20 percent, much more than the 1 to 4 percent forecast for the food industry overall.

So, what's the catch? In most cases, the health claims accompanying these products are based on flimsy or absent facts. Unfortunately, the industry seems to equate health claims with those promoting general products such as household cleansers, etc. We all know that such commercial claims are either wildly over hyped or simply bald-faced lies, but serious consequences seldom result from having a dingy floor or clothing that bears a faint shade of gray. Obviously, sloppy labeling does not carry over to issues of health.

Fortunately for all of us, the Food and Drug Administration (FDA) doesn't recognize functional food as an actual food category. As defined by the FDA's Federal Food, Drug, and Cosmetic Act, products with claims of treating specific diseases are considered to be drugs and therefore must meet the agency's rigorous regulatory requirements, including proof that they are safe and effective for their intended use. Thus if manufacturers wish to claim that its products have specific health-promoting properties, they must have credible science to back it up.

For example, the maker of POM Wonderful 100% Pomegranate Juice and POMx liquid supplement maintains that it has scientific proof to support the claim that its products prevent or treat heart disease, prostate cancer, and erectile dysfunction. Now anyone in his/her right mind must question the validity of such claims. Happily, the Federal Trade Commission (FTC) cracked down on the company for making what it calls false and unsubstantiated claims. "Any consumer who sees POM Wonderful products as a silver bullet against disease has been misled," says David Vladeck, director of the FTC's Bureau of Consumer Protection. "When a company touts scientific research in its advertising, the research must squarely support the claims made. Contrary to POM Wonderful's advertising, the available scientific information does not prove that POM Juice or POMx effectively treats or prevents these illnesses." In response, the company has filed a federal lawsuit contending that the agency is overstepping its authority by setting new standards for advertising food and dietary supplements. I seriously doubt that they can make much of a case.

In response to industrial lobbying for the right to promote the benefits of their products, Congress passed some ill-advised legislation: the Nutrition Labeling and Education Act forced the FDA to permit health claims on food packages, and in 1994 they passed the Dietary Supplement Health and Education Act, which made it easier to put health claims on vitamins, minerals, and herbal products.

"We expected to see nutritional supplements or dietary supplements making health claims," said Mary K. Engle, associate director of the FTC's Advertising Practices division. "But then, about five years ago, we started to see those kinds of claims on foods—claims like 'metabolism-enhancing' and 'immune-boosting,' or something having to do with brain health or heart health."

More recently, there have been claims about digestive health. For example, claims by Dannon that a daily serving of Activia yogurt could help with constipation caught the FTC's attention in 2010, and the agency accused the company of deceptive marketing practices. Dannon said it had scientific proof, but regulators concluded that many of its studies actually found that Activia was no more helpful than a placebo. Also, the probiotics (a type of healthful bacteria) in Activia might help digestion, but only if the yogurt is eaten three times a day—something not mentioned in the ads or on the packaging. Dannon eventually settled with the FTC, but admitted no wrong-doing.

What's A Health-Conscious Shopper to Do?

"Know thyself," says Elizabeth Rahavi, R.D., director of health and wellness at the International Food Information Council Foundation, an industry group. "Consumers can ask: 'Is this a food that I would commonly consume?' Often the benefit of a functional food comes through repeated consumption."

If any product—food, supplement, or otherwise—is accompanied by the following label: "This treatment has not been evaluated by the Food and Drug Administration. This product is not intended to diagnose, treat, cure, or prevent any disease," run the other direction; it is almost certainly a scam.

If you're still not sure about a given food, check the website of the Academy of Nutrition and Dietetics and the IFIC Foundation to see if a product's claims are backed up by credible research. And don't just read marketing claims; look at nutrition panels and ingredient lists.

Above all, always be skeptical and, whenever possible, avoid excessive expenditures.

CHAPTER 37

Genetically Modified (Gm) Foods and Mass Hysteria: The Facts

Whole Foods Market, the grocery chain, became the first retailer in the United States to begin to require labeling of all genetically modified (GM) foods sold in its stores. But was this move merely a marketing ploy to surround itself with an aura of "purity"? Since Whole Foods specializes in organic products that are less apt to be genetically modified, the company, in taking such a stance on labeling, is likely to capture increased market share from more traditional food retailers. The strategy by Whole Foods is one in a series of events that has intensified a debate over whether all foods should be required to be labeled as genetically modified.

Many Americans are suspicious about what they are eating and thus have requested that food from genetically modified (GM) crops be labeled as such, if not eliminated. Variable successes in this endeavor have been achieved at ballot boxes in several states. Going one step beyond mere labeling, Hawaii Island, in response to overwhelming public support, has banned even the cultivation of all genetically engineered crops on the island, with the exceptions of corn and papaya (which had already proved to be highly successful). The Food and Drug Administration is often urged to mandate such labeling for the entire country. Unfortunately, however, the general public is largely unaware of what a GM plant actually is and what advantages the technology has to offer. With regard to such crops, two main areas of concern have emerged:

1. Impact on human health.

2. Effects on the environment. Below I will examine these and other points and detail the considerable advantages possessed by these plants.

What are Genetically Modified Plant Foods?

Plants with favorable characteristics have been produced for thousands of years by conventional breeding methods. Desirable traits are selected, combined, and propagated by repeated crossings over multiple generations. This is a long process, taking up to 15 years to produce new varieties. Genetic engineering allows this process to be dramatically accelerated in a highly targeted manner.

Transgenic plants are those that have been genetically modified using recombinant DNA technology. This may involve including a gene that is not native to the plant or to modify existing genes capable of conferring a particular trait to that plant. The technology can be used in a number of ways, for example to create resistance to various stresses such as drought, extreme temperature or salinity, and resistance to harmful insects. It can also improve the nutritional content of the plant, an application that could be of particular use in the developing world. New-generation GM crops are now even being developed for the production of medicines and industrial products, such as antibodies, vaccines, plastics, and biofuels.

Food derived from GM plants is ubiquitous in the USA, and is also included in many animal feeds. Similarly, GM cotton is widely used in clothing and other products.

The Need for More Crops

In the developing world, 840 million people are chronically undernourished and do not have secure access to food. Many of them are also rural farmers in developing countries, depending entirely on small-scale agriculture for their own subsistence and for a livelihood. They generally cannot afford to irrigate their crops or purchase herbicides or pesticides, leading to poor crop growth, falling yields, and pest susceptibility. To meet the increased demands in a growing world, food production in the next few decades must increase substantially in the face of decreasing fertile lands and water resources. GM plant technologies are one of a number of different approaches that are being developed to combat these problems. Specifically, studies are under way to genetically modify plants both to increase crop yields and to improve nutritional content.

Commercial GM crops can be made to be insect resistant, a worldwide advantage. This has been particularly successful in the USA: For example, insect resistant GM corn is grown over millions of acres and comprises 35% of all corn grown in this country.

Insect-resistant GM cotton requires far less pesticide application and produces higher crop yields than the non-GM counterpart, generating savings of up to $200 per acre for farmers.

Increasing Nutritional Content

In the developed world the nutritional content of food items is not of major concern, as individuals have access to a wide variety of foods that will meet all of their nutritional needs. In the developing world, however, people often rely on a single staple food crop. GM technology offers a way to alleviate some of these problems by creating plants that can combat malnutrition.

An important example of the potential of this technology is the 'Golden Rice Project.' Vitamin A deficiency is widespread in the developing world and is estimated to account for the deaths of approximately 2 million children per year. In surviving children it has been identified as the leading cause of blindness. Humans can synthesize vitamin A from its precursor β-carotene, which is commonly found in many plants but not in cereal grains. The strategy of the Golden Rice Project was to introduce the correct metabolic steps into rice endosperm to allow β-carotene synthesis. In 2000, one group of scientists engineered rice that contained moderate levels of β-carotene, and since then other researchers have produced the much higher yielding 'Golden Rice 2.' It is estimated that about two ounces of dry Golden Rice 2 will provide 50% of the requirement of vitamin A for a one to three year-old child. This is an impressive example of a health solution that can be offered by plant biotechnology.

Are Gm Foods Safe to Eat?

For more than a decade, almost all processed foods in the United States—cereals, snack foods, salad dressings—have contained ingredients from plants whose DNA was manipulated in a laboratory. Regulators and scientists say these pose no danger.

In the USA, the Food and Drug Agency, the Environmental Protection Agency and the US Department of Agriculture, Animal and Plant Health Inspection Service are all involved in the regulatory process for GM crop approval. Consequently, GM plants undergo extensive and rigorous safety testing prior to commercialization.

Foods derived from GM crops have been consumed by hundreds of millions of people across the world for more than 15 years, with no reported ill effects (or legal cases related to human health), despite many of the consumers coming from that most litigious of countries, the USA.

Is there any reason that GM crops might be harmful when consumed? The presence of foreign DNA sequences in food *per se* poses no intrinsic risk to human health. All foods contain significant amounts of DNA. Of potential concern is the possibility that the protein produced by the modified gene may be toxic, but such a negative effect has not been found after careful safety assessment of these products.

A potential allergic response to the novel gene product is another commonly expressed concern. New varieties of crops produced by either GM techniques or conventional breeding both have the potential to cause allergies. Concern surrounding this topic relates to two factors; the possibility that genes from known allergens may be inserted into crops not typically associated with such problems and the possibility of creating new, unknown allergens by either inserting novel genes into crops or changing the expression of endogenous proteins. In response to this issue, scientists have devoted much effort in studying both humans and animals. Thus far, the allergic potential for such products appears to be less than—or equal to—their "naturally" grown counterparts. In some instances, safety testing of GM plants has been effective in identifying allergenic potential before some products have been released to market. By contrast, if conventional plant breeding techniques had been used to achieve the same aims, there would have been no legal requirement for the assessment of allergenicity, and the plant varieties could have been commercialized without any such testing. Moreover, GM technology might also be used to *decrease* the levels of allergens present in plants by reducing expression levels of the relevant genes. For example, research was recently undertaken to identify an allergen in soybeans and remove it using GM technology.

Gm Plants and the Environment

GM plants may potentially adversely affect human health for three reasons:

> 1.	They might form unfavorable hybrids with non-GM plants.

> 2.	They might themselves become invasive weeds.

> 3.	They might inadvertently harm local wildlife populations.

To date, none of these fears has materialized. By contrast, GM plants may have a positive role to play in the environment by selective removal of pollutants. For example, plants have already been genetically engineered to accumulate heavy metal soil contaminants such as mercury and selenium to higher levels than would be possible for non-GM plants, so not only can they grow on contaminated sites but they can also reduce contamination. These plants can be harvested and destroyed, the heavy metals disposed of or recycled, and the decontaminated field re-used.

Gm Plants and Public Opinion

According to a survey taken by the Pew Research Center, the differences in beliefs about this issue between the public and scientists are wide; 88% of scientists think GMO foods are safe, whereas only 37% of the American public think they are safe.

Several organizations are implacably opposed to GM plants. Crops that have been designed to help relieve malnutrition in the developing world, such as Golden Rice, are attacked on the basis that it "tastes awful" and that "to be of any benefit a child would have to eat approximately 3 lbs of cooked Golden Rice," an over-estimation by more than 15 times according to best estimates.

Others have irrationally claimed GM food is "unnatural," despite the fact that all our food has been produced over millennia by artificial breeding. When considering "natural" food production, one should recognize that technology has always played an important role in this enterprise and will continue to do so.

Opposition to GM crops is fairly widespread, possibly attributable to the public's current infatuation with "unadulterated" or "organic" products, despite the fact that food from GM crops already comprises a large portion of the normal diet in this country.

Nevertheless, since much opposition to GM crops does exist, scientists must work to combat the misinformation and biases that exist. Persistent opposition is having many serious effects, especially because many developing countries that could benefit from the technology will not take it up as long as they believe that there remain significant areas of concern and that their potential for exports will be seriously impaired. This then reduces opportunities for improving GM crops to provide a solution that will be crucial in helping to alleviate current and future challenges in food and medicine supply.

Conclusion:

Forcing the industry to label or eliminate GM foods not only sends the wrong message, suggesting that these foods somehow are "impure." This makes about as much sense as forcing them to state that oatmeal contains "oats" or that popcorn contains "corn." Irrational opposition to these products is likely being propagated by the same individuals who deny, among others, global warming and evolution.

CHAPTER 38

Should You Consider Buying and Consuming Organic Foods?

The popularity of organic products is skyrocketing in the United States. Between 1997 and 2011, U.S. sales of organic foods increased from $3.6 billion to $24.4 billion, and many consumers are willing to pay a premium for these products. Organic foods are generally grown without synthetic pesticides or fertilizers or routine use of antibiotics or growth hormones, and they are often twice as expensive as their conventionally grown counterparts. For instance, you're in the supermarket eyeing a basket of sweet, juicy plums. You reach for the conventionally grown fruit, and then decide to pony up the extra $1/pound for its organic cousin. You figure you've just made the healthier decision by choosing the organic product. But have you? This is a common perception — perhaps based on this high price, or simply on one's naturalistic fantasies—that organic foods are better for you than the conventional ones.

In order to provide some guidance, a recent extensive review of this subject was provided by a team from Stanford University[58]. They evaluated a large number of existing studies comparing organic and conventional foods.

In their study the researchers sifted through thousands of scientific publications and identified 237 of the most relevant to analyze. Those included 17 studies (six of which were randomized clinical trials) of populations consuming organic and conventional diets, and 223 studies that compared either the nutrient levels or the bacterial, fungal or pesticide contamination of various products (fruits, vegetables, grains, meats, milk, poultry, and eggs) grown organically and conventionally. There were no long-term studies of health outcomes of people consuming organic versus conventionally produced food; the duration of the studies involving human subjects ranged from two days to two years.

After analyzing the data, the researchers found no significant difference in health benefits between organic and conventional foods. No consistent differences were seen in the vitamin content of organic products, and only one nutrient — phosphorus — was significantly higher in organic versus conventionally grown produce (and the researchers noted that because few people have phosphorous deficiency, this had little impact on health). There was also no difference in protein or fat content between organic and conventional milk, though evidence from a limited number of studies suggested that organic milk may contain higher levels of omega-3 fatty acids, a finding also of questionable health benefit.

The review yielded scant evidence that conventional foods posed greater health risks than organic products. While researchers found that organic produce had a 30 percent lower risk of pesticide contamination than conventional fruits and vegetables, organic foods are not necessarily 100 percent free of pesticides. What's more, as the researchers noted, the pesticide levels of all foods generally fell within the allowable safety limits. Two studies of children consuming organic and conventional diets did find lower levels of pesticide residues in the urine of children on organic diets, though the significance of these findings on child health was also unclear. Additionally, organic chicken and pork appeared to reduce exposure to antibiotic-resistant bacteria, but the clinical significance of this again is questionable.

So what can we conclude from all this? First, there is no real evidence that organic foods are more nutritious than conventional foods. If your taste buds are highly sensitive and you can discern a better flavor with organic foods (most people can't), then go ahead and buy—provided you can afford it! On the other hand, there is no convincing proof that minor increases in pesticide or chemical residuals in conventional food are an actual threat to health, but long-term studies should help to provide more definitive information. In the meantime, you can minimize the risks of such contamination by simply carefully washing off conventional foods prior to preparing and serving them at the table.

CHAPTER 39

Gluten-Free Diets: A Mistake for Most Folks

A decade ago, few Americans had heard of gluten. Today, one survey has found that almost a third of our population is trying to avoid this component found in grain. In growing numbers, the world's biggest food makers and restaurant chains are retooling recipes and labels to tap into that concern, creating a multibillion-dollar business out of gluten-free products. They have churned out a bevy of new foods and eating initiatives, producing a whole new fad. And predictably, food companies are charging as much as double for some of these "better-for-you" products, keeping profit margins healthier than the contents of those foods they are offering.

But, for most of us, joining the gluten craze is pure claptrap! There is no proven benefit to going gluten-free except for an estimated 1% to 2% of the population whose bodies can't process the protein. Worse yet, according to nutritional food labels, many gluten-free foods contain fewer vitamins, less fiber, and more sugar. It is a point some food makers don't dispute, saying they are simply responding to consumer demand without making health claims.

What is Gluten?

Gluten is a protein found in wheat, barley and rye. Its elastic structure makes it well-suited for baking. But it can produce a condition called "celiac disease," which is believed due to an autoimmune inflammatory response in the lining of the small intestines The symptoms include abdominal cramping, diarrhea, anemia, bone pain, and, occasionally, a severe skin rash. Rarely celiac disease may have few symptoms, but under these circumstances, benign conditions such as irritable bowel syndrome are usually responsible.

A gluten-free diet excludes this protein, and as a result, can control the signs and symptoms of celiac disease. But how can you know if you have celiac disease? The only sure way is to be tested. But if you have minor symptoms suggesting this disorder, you could first try eliminating gluten, and if symptoms are completely relieved, stick with this program. If not, the first test is typically a blood test that detects antibodies related to an abnormal immune response. If the blood test is positive, a biopsy can be performed to confirm inflammation in the lining of the small intestines.

Unfortunately, in most cases, removing gluten from baked goods, noodles, and other products is difficult. Wheat substitutes don't retain fat or hold their structure as well, and many taste really bad. Wheat flour is typically enriched with vitamins and minerals, while many of the specialty flours used in gluten-free products aren't. Moreover, many gluten-free products are loaded with sugar and other unhealthy ingredients. Fortunately, some gluten-free products are nutritionally the same as their gluten-containing counterparts. The nutritional composition of Chex cereal, for example, didn't change when General Mills removed the gluten.

Another concern centers on the plethora of gluten-free snacks and desserts that exists today. Ten years ago a gluten-free diet would have helped you lose weight because you'd have cut out a lot of products like muffins and bread. Paradoxically, the gluten-free fad has actually undermined people's health because now there are gluten-free varieties of all kinds of junk food. So don't try to be gluten free in order to lose weight.

If You Must Go On a Gluten-Free Diet

Switching to a gluten-free diet is a big change and, like anything new, it takes some getting used to. You may initially feel deprived by the diet's restrictions. However, stay positive and focus on all the foods you can eat. You may also be pleasantly surprised to realize how many gluten-free products, such as bread and pasta, are now available. Many specialty grocery stores sell gluten-free foods. If you can't find them in your area, check with a celiac support group or go online.

If you're just starting with a gluten-free diet, it's a good idea to consult a dietitian who can answer your questions and offer advice about how to avoid gluten while still eating a healthy, balanced diet. Specific lists of gluten free foods can be found on the Mayo Clinic Website: http://www.mayoclinic.org/healthy-living/nutrition-and-healthy-eating/in-depth/gluten-free-diet/art-20048530

Conclusion:

If you are basically healthy and have no significant recurring gastrointestinal distress, don't go gluten-free. It's a waste of money.

CHAPTER 40

Bottled Water: Another Great—and Costly—Myth!

Global bottled water sales have increased dramatically over the past several decades. The rate of consumption more than quadrupled between 1990 and 2005. "Spring water" and "purified tap water" are currently the leading global sellers. By one estimate, approximately 50 billion bottles of water are consumed per annum in the U.S. and around the world, 200 billion bottles.

But does this huge rush into these products make sense? Should we ignore tap water? First let's look at safety issues. I'll leave the taste issues up to you.

Is Tap Water Safe?

Tap water contents can vary greatly depending upon where you live. The EPA oversees municipal water supplies, and one way to find out what's in your water is to check your consumer confidence report, or CCR. The EPA requires utilities to provide a CCR to their customers every year. You may also find the CCR printed in your newspaper or posted on your local government website. A recent analysis of CCRs from the 13 largest U.S. cities revealed that few claimed to have no federal water-quality violations. All had some samples containing significant quantities of contaminants. In

New York City, for example, some samples had lead levels several times the federal limit. A CCR might indicate safe levels of a contaminant when your water actually has experienced potentially harmful temporary spikes. Also, a CCR tells you about the water in your municipality, but not necessarily about what's coming out of your own tap. Only testing your home supply can do that. Homeowners with a well on their property face even greater uncertainty, because such water isn't surveyed or reported on in CCRs. For that information, call the EPA's Safe Drinking Water Hotline (800-426-4791) for the names of state-certified testing labs or for your local health authority, which might offer low-cost or free test kits, or check out www.epa.gov/safewater/labs. Ultimately, you might find that your water is safe and can be consumed without alteration.

It's important to know that, if contaminants are in your water, you can take proper defensive measures, often involving the acquisition of a filter. From a funny taste to lead contamination from aging pipes, your tap water may have picked up some unsavory additions along the way. If you are concerned, have your water tested by a lab that's certified by the state; the EPA has an online listing of certification officers, or call your health department for recommendations. If you determine that a filter is required, claims about contaminant removal by those selling filters vary from product to product, so read the fine print. Also, consider how much water you consume vs. how much effort and disruption to your daily routine you're willing to tolerate. Generally, the more contaminants you need to remove, the more complicated the filter, though there are trade-offs. For a comprehensive review of filters, I suggest you consult with consumer reports:

www.consumerreports.org/cro/health/index.htm.

Choices range from tabletop containers, such as a carafe with a carbon filter, to devices that purify the water as it enters your home. In between are faucet-mounted, under-sink, and reverse osmosis units. Look for one approved by NSF, Underwriters Laboratories or the Water Quality Association, and clean it as recommended by the manufacturer. Some water is treated with chlorine to kill bacteria, but the taste often turns people off. The fix? Pour water into a clear glass container and leave it uncovered in the refrigerator for 24 hours to let the chlorine dissipate into the air. Bottled water may be your only other choice.

Notwithstanding these comments, most municipal water is quite safe, and if palatable, can be taken directly from the tap. It often contains the useful minerals, magnesium and calcium. As you will find in chapter 41, soft water for drinking should generally be avoided because of the addition of sodium, which is undesirable.

Bottled Water

The Food and Drug Administration (FDA) oversees bottled water, while the Environmental Protection Agency (EPA) regulates tap water. However, both use similar standards for ensuring safety.

The FDA has good manufacturing practices specifically for bottled water. They require bottled water producers to:

1. Process, bottle, hold, and transport bottled water under sanitary conditions

2. Protect water sources from bacteria, chemicals, and other contaminants

3. Use quality control processes to ensure the bacteriological and chemical safety of the water

4. Sample and test both source water and the final product for contaminants

Despite the aggressive marketing, however, bottled water is generaly not safer than tap water. Since bottled water is regulated by the Food and Drug Administration, this agency is perpetually under-funded and short-staffed, and, therefore, has a poor record of protecting consumer health and safety. FDA sends inspectors to bottling plants once every two to three years.

Some Facts about Bottled Water

1.   In 2009, almost 50 percent of all bottled water came from municipal tap water supplies.

2.   According to a 2010 survey, only 3 companies provided the public with the same level of information available for tap water. This includes where the water came from, how it was treated and what the results of the water quality tests were.

3.   Independent testing of bottled water conducted by the Environmental Working Group in 2008 found that 10 popular brands of bottled water, purchased from grocery stores and other retailers in 9 states and the District of Columbia, contained 38 chemical pollutants, with an average of 8 contaminants in each brand.

Fluoride Facts

Most bottled water doesn't contain added fluoride (if it does, it will say so on the label). Kids are drinking more bottled water and less fluoridated from the tap, and some say that's behind the recent rise in dental decay. Thus choosing bottled water without fluoride loses an opportunity to protect children's teeth from decay. If your tap water contains fluoride and you don't use a filter, stick with that source for your major drinking water supply. If your family has well water without fluoride, is drinking only bottled water or using a filter that removes fluoride (many do), ask your dentist about supplements for your child.

But The Bottled Water Story Gets Even Worse

Plastic bottles are made from petroleum. Energy is required to manufacture the bottles and run the bottling and refrigeration machines. It also requires fuel, typically petro-diesel, to transport the bottles to the place where you buy them. These combined energy costs are the oil equivalent of about one quarter the volume of each bottle and 1000 times greater than the energy costs to pump, treat, and deliver tap water. This explains why bottled water is far more expensive and wasteful than tap water.

The production process for a bottle of water wastes the equivalent of about 3 or 4 bottles of tap water. Also, many plastic bottles are not properly sorted for recycling and end up as litter or non-biodegradable trash, bound for a landfill or waste incinerator.

So What Should You Do?

From this information, the answer should be obvious, but here are my recommendations:

1.   **Reject Bottled Water: Stick with the Tap.** First, check out your own water supply, as indicated above. It's usually quite safe.

2.   **Get a Canteen.** If you wish to carry water, put your plain or filtered tap water in a reusable stainless steel or lined drinking container, and clean it between uses. Some come with an easy-to-tote strap.

3.   **Think Twice about the Office Water Cooler.** If it's made of polycarbonate, it has the potential to leach BPA, a chemical that can cause neurological problems, among other things. And have

you ever seen anyone actually clean the water cooler? Probably not.

4. **_Shop Smart._** When you must have bottled water, look for brands that have NSF certification or belong to IBWA. Check out the lists at nsf.org or bottledwater.org, or look at the bottle itself (the NSF logo appears on labels of tested brands). If the brand you're looking for isn't there, contact the bottler. Ask where the water is bottled and what exactly is in it.

5. **_Keep It Cool._** Don't drink from a bottle that's been subjected to high temperatures (sitting in your car, for example), don't store it anywhere it will be exposed to heat or chemicals, and don't reuse plastic bottles.

6. **_Go With Glass._** Choose glass containers (Eden Springs and Voss are two popular brands) over plastic whenever possible. When you're done, recycle!

CHAPTER 41

Myths about Hard and Soft Water

Most folks think hard water is bad in general and it should be replaced by soft water. The "softening" process is usually accomplished by applying various chemical agents to hard water.

But what causes water to be "hard"? Most water from public sources and wells is considered hard because it contains variable amounts of calcium and magnesium. Both of these minerals are classed as "contaminants," but that's a poor choice of words, for calcium is essential in our diet, and magnesium is also helpful. Although these minerals promote hard deposits on plumbing equipment and interfere with cleansing of dishes and clothing, drinking hard water might promote better health, as I explain below.

In most water softening devices, hard water flows through synthetic resin beads. Sodium ions (salt) are loosely attached to each bead and the water exchanges hardness ions (calcium and magnesium) for sodium ions. Thus soft water contains variable amounts of sodium, a mineral that may pose a threat to health by elevating the blood pressure, or at least causing more difficulty in managing this problem if present. In areas with very hard water, the process of softening water coming from your tap can actually add a significant amount of sodium to your diet. The harder the water, the more sodium the softening system must add to replace the dissolved calcium and magnesium. In order to figure out how much sodium your softener is adding, your local health department can usually tell you how hard your water is. Generally the hardness of your water is expressed in "grains per gallon." You can multiply this number by 8 to find out how much sodium (expressed in milligrams per liter) will be added to your water by your water softener. In general, typical softened water contains about 12.5mg of sodium per 8oz glass. If this water were graded according to the same scale the Food and Drug Administration uses for foods, it would be considered "very low sodium." But if you live in an area with very hard water, or tend to drink a lot of tap water, this extra sodium can start to add up. Studies have shown that significantly decreasing sodium intake can lower your blood pressure by an appreciable amount (Chapter 13).

Emerging evidence suggests that hard water may prevent cardiovascular disease, at least in comparison with soft water. A recent study in the International Journal of Preventive Medicine[59], deriving data from the years 2010 and 2011, water calcium content above 72 mg/L was associated with reduced number of cardiovascular events per 1000 population. The level of water magnesium content ranged from 23 to 57 mg/L. By increasing magnesium levels above 31 mg/L in 2010 and above 26 mg/L in 2011, decreased cardiovascular events were recorded. The researchers concluded that, in all likelihood, water hardness, mainly water magnesium content, could prevent or reduce cardiovascular disease. Although these results agreed with earlier studies, further experimental studies are necessary to determine the underlying mechanisms, and studies over longer time intervals are required to study the clinical impacts of these findings.

How should the individual react to this information? Drinking hard water should be encouraged in preference to soft water, especially if the latter is high in sodium content. This might be facilitated most easily by hooking up water softeners only to the hot water source, which is used for washing but not drinking, or you may want to consider a water-purification system that uses potassium instead of sodium.

CHAPTER 42

Wifi: Mythical and Unfounded Fears

There appear to be growing and unfounded fears about the supposed health dangers of wireless networking (Wifi). Although most recently involving Canada, the same myths have also affected the U.S., where fear mongers are easily found to roil up the population with all kinds of nutty theories. Recently, across Canada anti-Wifi activists are spreading misinformation about Wifi and related technologies, blaming these networks' low level radio signals for a broad variety of medical problems, from mild headaches and fatigue to chest pain and heart palpitations, claiming those who suffer from them have "Electromagnetic-Hypersensitivity," or EHS. These kinds of claims periodically arise in the U.S., ranging from fear of brain tumors in those using cell phones, to scares of contracting malignancies in those residing near high-voltage power lines.

None of these claims have ever been substantiated by scientific study and have little acceptance from medical professionals such as myself, and the scientific community at large. This activism therefore usually amounts to nothing more than fear-mongering by special interest groups who are attempting to have these networks removed. Nevertheless, in Canada at least, the media has been all too willing to fan the flames of controversy and has contributed to a growing false uncertainty over the safety of Wifi. As a result many school boards, libraries, and town councils across that country have been called on by fearful citizens to limit or remove Wifi networks.

Those who stand the most to suffer from these efforts are students (especially from low-income families) who rely on wireless networks for access to the internet and education resources, and taxpayers who will have to pay for the expensive reversion to wired networks. In addition, families are being misled into believing that their children are suffering from EHS and may actually miss an opportunity for early diagnosis of real and serious health problems in their children.

Unfortunately, many of these activists have financial motives aimed to profit from the fear-mongering by offering products to 'block' Wifi signals. Examples of such products include electromagnetic field shielding curtains and screens, wallpaper, clothing, even 21st century equivalents of tin-foil hats. Particularly disturbing are the people promoting quack diagnoses and treatments for EHS.

But above all, don't get caught up in this nonsense. Those who desire further information about this problem may find it at the following location: BSW Anti-Wifi 2012 Position Paper Updated Jan 27 2013.

CHAPTER 43

Hand Drying: Paper Towels or Blower?

Have you ever wondered whether there was really any advantage in blow-drying your hands in the washroom? After all, there must be some compensation—other than saving money for the innkeeper—for the prolonged wait necessary for drying one's hands in a public restroom. Even after that interminably long delay, however, I usually must finish hand drying with a handkerchief or other handy cloth item anyway. Nevertheless, intuition tells us that this method should clearly be the most hygienic method—right? Guess again—wrong!

Well, fear not my friends; a reasonable answer to this question has recently been provided in a study generated by researchers at the Mayo Clinic[60].

This group reviewed the available evidence regarding speed of drying, extent of dryness, effective removal of bacteria, and prevention of cross-contamination. Most studies they reviewed concluded similarly that paper towels can dry hands sufficiently, remove bacteria effectively, and cause less contamination of the washroom environment. From a hygienic viewpoint, therefore, paper towels are superior to electric blow-dryers. This group concluded that paper towels should be recommended in locations where hygiene is paramount, such as hospitals and clinics. Although that seems counter-intuitive, facts are facts.

So, what is the best overall procedure in the washroom? First, thorough washing should be accomplished with soap and water. Disinfectant soaps are probably of no advantage. Drying, as noted, is best done with paper towels. Blowers are less effective, probably because, if used for less than one minute, the hands remain damp, and wetness promotes the presence of residual bacteria. Moreover, a blower may promote dissemination of bacteria to the neighboring environment enhancing the chances for cross-contamination. Finally, the least desirable method of drying is with the cloth roller towels, which are a source of contaminants, especially when the end of the roll accommodates more than one user.

From a personal standpoint, I would recommend paper towels everywhere. This method might even provide an economic boost to our lumber industry.

An additional and related risk concerns the flushing of open toilets, which can release toxic microbes, both bacteria and viruses, into the immediate vicinity[61,62]. Many individuals are unaware of the risk of air-borne dissemination of microbes by flushing toilets and the consequent surface and air contamination that may spread infection. Risky microorganisms may persist in the air after toilet flushing, and infection may be acquired from air inhalation or surface contact. In order to minimize this risk, one must close the toilet lid before flushing. In the process, this closure also prevents an individual's remaining on the commode during the flushing process, which can contaminate the skin from the same source.

From this information, the message is clear: Whether at home or away, first get off the commode, then close the lid, and then, finally—flush.

CHAPTER 44

Probiotics and Health: A Mixed Bag—Facts And Myths

Most people are aware of the allegedly new health "miracles" called probiotics. Promoters claim that they help with a variety of health problems, ranging from constipation to diarrhea, preventing and fighting colds, the strengthening of the immune system, the improvement of the skin's function, the strengthening of the resistance to cedar pollen allergens, the protection of DNA, and the combating of many other maladies. As a result, probiotics are showing up widely in foods, beverages, and supplements.

So what are probiotics? The root of the word probiotic comes from the Greek word pro, meaning "promoting" and biotic, meaning "life." Many experts define probiotics as live microorganisms, which, when administered in adequate amounts, potentially confer a health benefit on the host. Most of these microorganisms are bacteria, but in this case they are "good" bacteria, not the ones that may cause infections.

Our digestive system normally contains a combination of billions of "good" bacteria and "bad" bacteria. Maintaining the correct balance between these two types of microorganisms is believed by many to be necessary for optimal health, primarily by holding bad actors in check and, in the process, promoting the correct balance between them. Things like medications, diet, diseases, and environment can upset this balance. In most studies thus far, however, the medical benefits of probiotics have yet to be conclusively demonstrated.

But there is at least one exception to this uncertainty: In recent years, certain intestinal infections are increasing, especially among people who are receiving antibiotics or who spend time in health care settings. Caused by the bacterium (germ) Clostridium difficile, often called "C. diff," this infection causes chronic diarrhea, abdominal pain, and intestinal inflammation, which, if very severe, can be fatal. Although it may occasionally infect those in the general population, it is especially prone to occur in individuals receiving antibiotics, which kill off large numbers of those beneficial bacteria residing in the intestines that are normally responsible for protecting us against these evil doers that are resistant to conventional antibiotics. Growing evidence indicates that preserving the trillions of good microorganisms in our intestines can defend us from this disease. Thus if we could provide these good bacteria, we may be able to combat at least this one serious intestinal infection. These bacteria are found in the form of probiotics, i.e., products that supply the live microbes that have been tested in human studies and found to be effective. They can be found in many foods and supplements, and manufacturers are adding probiotics to all sorts of products, from trail mix to chocolate bars. More targeted products such as DanActive dairy drink, and pills and packets of powder with brand names such as BioK Plus, Culturelle, Florastor, and VSL#3. Culturelle, a supplement containing Lactobacillus rhamnosus GG (LGG), is gushingly claimed; "to promote digestion, maintain regularity, support your immune system, and help you return to optimal health." Unlike a lot of probiotics, a Culturelle spokeswoman notes,

LGG survives past the stomach and into the intestines, where it "balances out bad bacteria." Each capsule is guaranteed to contain 10 billion cells of LGG. Because probiotics are considered a dietary supplement rather than a medicine, the Food and Drug Administration doesn't verify their claims. But many strains of probiotic bacteria have been studied extensively for their effect on irritable bowel syndrome, eczema, and diarrhea. Consumer reports recently reviewed LGG studies, looking for evidence to support or refute these various claims. They concluded that, although no studies have been very large and are inconclusive, some hold promise for travelers, people taking antibiotics, or kids with diarrhea, as noted below:

1. A 1997 study of 245 adults who took LGG or placebo to prevent diarrhea when traveling to various countries showed that those who took LGG cut diarrhea risk almost in half.

2. A 1999 study of LGG's ability to prevent or lessen antibiotic-associated diarrhea in children found that 26 percent who took placebo had diarrhea, compared with 8 percent who took LGG.

3. A 2000 study involving 287 youngsters from 10 countries found that LGG reduced infectious diarrhea by a day compared with placebo.

Certain natural foods such as yogurt also contain probiotic lactobacilli and others, and they possess similar potential advantages for the digestive disorders noted above. Our knowledge is limited, however, about which yogurt brands, if any, might be most effective for this purpose. Below we list a few general comments:

Know the dose and type: Large numbers of viable organisms are likely best suited to achieve benefits. Colony forming units, or CFUs, represents the measure of viable microorganisms in a probiotic. The level of CFUs likely to yield benefit differs by probiotic, ranging from 50 million to more than 500 billion per day. In general, yogurts are the most power packed products, containing from 90 billion to 500 billion CFUs per serving. Various dietary supplements contain less, ranging from under 1 billion to 20 billion per capsule. Certain snack foods such as chocolate bars and trail mixes also are said to contain varying numbers, but are generally fewer in quantity and also tend to possess more calories than desirable for the possible gains promoted. To reduce the risk of diarrhea caused by C. diff, the most effective dose is believed to be more than 10 billion CFUs per day. When considering yogurt brands, look for the National Yogurt Associations Live and Active Cultures seal that tells you that the given product contains at least 100 million live cultures per gram at the time of manufacture.

Research suggests that the most effective probiotics are combinations of L. acidophilus, L. casei, L. rhaminosus, and S boulardii.

Beware of expiration dates. Probiotics contain live microorganisms and may lose their effectiveness after a certain date. Some probiotics require refrigeration to preserve the active ingredients. Dairy products, specifically, tend to have a short shelf life. One should follow handling and storage instructions on the package.

Make sure it's from a trusted source. Check the product website to determine if the manufacturer is reputable and review the evidence base for a given product.

Keep in mind that continued administration is necessary for probiotics to be beneficial in the gastrointestinal tract. Also look for labels that say "live active cultures," as many prepackaged and processed foods, including even some yogurt brands, contain few to no viable bacteria.

More research may help clarify the proper dosage and strains for different conditions. Meanwhile, probiotics aren't useful to everyone. Basically, if you are a healthy person and maintain a healthy way of life and healthy diet, you don't need probiotics to help you get healthier.

Research also shows that the need for probiotics may depend on the person's situation. It may be advisable for those that are prone to antibiotic associated diarrhea to try probiotics, at least during and a few days after taking the antibiotic. However, further study clearly is needed to determine which specific probiotics should be tried and who precisely should try them.

Overall, various conditions are at least potentially amenable to a trial of probiotics are as listed below:

1. Treating diarrhea – both the infectious kind and that which occurs as a result of the use of antibiotics

2. Reducing the symptoms of conditions such as irritable bowel syndrome and inflammatory bowel conditions such as Crohn's disease and ulcerative colitis

3. Decreasing lactose intolerance

4. Lowering cholesterol levels

5. Reducing or preventing high blood pressure

6. Treating constipation

As this list above suggests, the entire subject is incredibly complex and speculative because of the number of variables involved, including the differing varieties of probiotic microorganisms. At present, although many avenues are being explored, research extends most notably to possible links between probiotics and heart attacks and effects on elevated blood pressure, but substantive results likely lie far in the future.

In summary then, although much research has yet to be done, if you are suffering from any of the conditions listed above, these products may be worth a try. Perhaps the best initial choice, however, is probiotic yogurt, because it is inexpensive, nutritious, and consuming it periodically certainly won't hurt.

Several sources of accurate information on probiotics are the American Gastroenterological Association, the International Scientific Association for Probiotics and Prebiotics and the FDA's website on dietary supplements.

C✑CHAPTER 45✑⁓

Raw Milk: Buyer Beware!

In this country there is a mythical—but accelerating—belief that raw milk is somehow superior to the pasteurized version.

Pasteurization, which is the process of heating of milk to destroy disease-causing bacteria, has been standard practice in the US since 1924 under the oversight of the Food and Drug Administration (FDA). Since 1987 the FDA has prohibited the interstate shipment of raw, unpasteurized, milk for human consumption. Nevertheless, sale of raw milk is permitted in 24 states, and in the remaining 26, where these sales are not allowed, various "gaming" schemes make such milk available to the consumer. These include selling raw milk labeled as "animal or pet food" across state lines, publishing lists of states where the sale of raw milk is allowed, and selling "shares" in cows or "leasing" cows. In states where sale of raw milk is legal, regulations vary—some allow sales in retail outlets and others restrict these sales to farm outlets directly to consumers.

With the advent of mandatory pasteurization, the incidence of milk borne diseases has fallen dramatically. In the US in 1938, contaminants in milk accounted for approximately 25% of all disease outbreaks traceable to food and water. By the year 2000, milk products were associated with less than 1% of all such outbreaks. However, the CDC has determined that consumption of raw milk or cheese from 1998 through 2009 accounted for 93 instances of disease, resulting in 1,837 illnesses, 195 hospitalizations, and 2 deaths, strongly implicating these products as a continued important public health concern. Although the very young, the aged, and immunocompromised persons (those harboring immunity-reducing conditions) are the most susceptible to the microbes that may be present in raw milk, anyone can be affected, including healthy young adults, as indicated by a recent outbreak of infection among 19 of 31 college students who consumed unpasteurized milk after a visit to a farm.

Despite such robust information to the contrary, certain organizations such as the Weston A. Price Foundation actively promote the legalization of raw milk, claiming that it is not only completely safe, but can prevent and treat a wide spectrum of diseases, including heart disease, kidney disease, cancer, lactose intolerance, allergies and eczema. None of these claims has ever been supported by scientific evidence. Also, despite opinions to the contrary, scientific studies uniformly indicate that pasteurization does not change the nutritional value of milk

As a result of efforts touting the supposed benefits of "unaltered organic" products, general demand for raw milk has increased greatly in recent years. According to the US Center for Disease Control and Prevention's Food Net Population Survey in 2002, 3.5% of respondents reported to have consumed unpasteurized milk in the preceding 7 days. And, not surprisingly, consumption of raw milk has always been common among farm families, currently running in the range of 50%.

When the public is presented with a large body of conflicting claims and counter claims, their decision-making process often does not equal that of the experts. The public is seldom privy to solid evidence, and is often easily seduced by anecdotal information, personal testimonials, and by strong, misleading statements by advocates.

In view of all this misleading "noise" I would simply reiterate the old cliché, *buyer beware!* I suspect that if he could be made aware of this nonsense today, the man who pioneered such milk cleansing in the 1880's that now bears his name, Louis Pasteur, would issue a mighty groan and probably utter (udder?) some expletives as well!

ᘓᔎCHAPTER 46ᕲᕲ

Radiation of Foods: Safe or Unsafe?

Food irradiation is a technology for controlling spoilage and eliminating food borne germs. The result is similar to pasteurization. The fundamental difference between food irradiation and pasteurization is the source of the energy used to destroy the microbes. While conventional pasteurization relies on heat, irradiation relies on the energy of ionizing radiation, which is a process in which approved foods are exposed to radiant energy, including gamma rays, electron beams, and x-rays. In 1963, the Food and Drug Administration (FDA) found the irradiation of food to be safe. Irradiation of meat and poultry is done in a government-approved irradiation facility. Such treatment is not a substitute for good sanitation in meat and poultry plants. It is simply an added layer of safety.

Notwithstanding common fears and misconceptions, food irradiation does not make foods radioactive. The radiant energy passes through the food. The food itself never contacts the source of the radiant energy. Irradiated foods are wholesome and nutritious. Nutrient losses caused by this process are less than or about the same as losses caused by cooking and freezing. Public health agencies worldwide have evaluated the safety of food irradiation over the last fifty years and found it to be safe. In 37 countries more than 40 food products are irradiated. In some European countries, irradiation has been in use for decades. In the United States, the Food and Drug Administration regulates food irradiation. In addition, food irradiation has received official endorsement from the American Medical Association, the World Health Organization, and the International Atomic Energy Agency.

The FDA first approved the use of irradiation in 1963 to kill pests in wheat and flour. Since then they have approved food irradiation for use on fruits, vegetables, spices, raw poultry, and red meats.

Consumers cannot recognize irradiated food by sight, smell, taste, or feel. Irradiated foods can be recognized by the presence of the international symbol for irradiation on the packaging along with the words "Treated with Radiation," or "Treated by Irradiation." If irradiated meat is used in another product, such as pork sausage, then the ingredients statement must list irradiated pork. Restaurants are not required to disclose the use of irradiated products to their customers; however, some restaurants voluntarily provide such information on menus—a meaningless gesture at best.

Despite its safety, food irradiation is not a substitute for good sanitation and does not replace safe cooking and handling. Consumers should handle irradiated foods just like any other food and always follow safe food handling practices. Inasmuch as labeling of such foods is unnecessary, if you encounter this moniker, it need not conjure up an image of Chernobyl or Three Mile Island. Conversely, you should feel that it possesses added safety, much the same as that of "Pasteurized" milk.

CHAPTER 47

Allergies: Myths Exposed

Misconceptions about allergies are rampant, and below I discuss some of the most common:

Myth: *Some Pets May Be "Hypo-Allergenic"*

Fact: Unfortunately, our dogs and cats are a common source of allergies; however, none are free of these problems, despite much advertising to the contrary. Approximately 10 to 15 percent of the population suffers from pet allergies. The allergen is a specific protein produced not in the animal's fur, but primarily in its skin and—a lesser extent—urine and saliva. As the animal is petted or brushed, or as it rubs up against furniture or people, microscopic flakes of skin (called dander) become airborne. Since all cats and dogs have skin, all are potentially allergenic. There's a lot of false advertising by companies marketing supposedly hypo-allergenic pets, some selling cats or dogs for as much as $7,000 or more. While some of these animals have been bred to produce fewer major allergens from their saliva, sebaceous glands, or other glands, they still produce allergens that cause unpleasant symptoms in sensitized people.

Since short-haired pets have less hair to shed, they send less dander into the air, so are probably preferable for those with pet allergies. Dogs are half as likely to cause allergic reactions as cats, but if you're allergic to furry animals, the only no-risk pets are fish and reptiles.

Myth: Allergies are Psychosomatic

Fact: Allergies are very real—in some cases, potentially life-threatening, rooted in heredity and the environment; yet the mind plays a significant role in their behavior. Mental stress can precipitate or enhance allergic reactions, and relaxation techniques can moderate them. A person who is strongly allergic to roses, for example, may react to the sight of a plastic rose, demonstrating the involvement of the mind and the brain, but this relationship is not well understood.

Myth: Blood Testing is a Good Way to Detect Allergies

Fact: Allergen-specific serum testing (for IgE) is not a reliable screen for allergy, and often leads to misinterpretation and false-positive results—which in turn lead to diagnostic confusion and unnecessarily eliminating foods from a diet. A negative test provides more useful evidence against such an allergy, but it also is not failsafe.

Myth: Skin Testing for Allergy is Unreliable

Fact: The idea that skin testing is unreliable until 2, 3, or 5 years of age is sheer myth, but an ongoing one. Most evidence indicates that skin testing is reliable at any age.

A positive result, i.e., a red, raised area called a wheal, means you reacted to a substance in a potentially allergic way. Such a positive result means the symptoms you are having are likely due to exposure to that substance. In general, the stronger the response, the greater the chance of allergy to that given substance.

Skin tests are usually accurate, although people can have a positive response to skin testing without any problems with that given substance in everyday life. On the other hand, if the dose of allergen applied to the skin is large, a positive reaction may occur in people who are not allergic. A negative test result means there were no skin changes in response to the allergen, and that usually means that you are not allergic to that substance. Rarely, however, a person may have a negative skin test and still be allergic to the substance. In general, allergy skin tests are most reliable for diagnosing allergies to airborne substances, such as pollen, pet dander, and dust mites. Skin testing may help diagnose food allergies. But because food allergies can be complex, you may need additional tests or procedures.

Your health care provider will consider your symptoms, considering the results of your skin test, to suggest lifestyle changes you can make to avoid substances that may be causing your symptoms.

Myth: No Milk, Eggs, or Nuts For Babies

Fact: Changes in recommendations over the years have contributed to the myth that highly allergenic food such as milk, eggs, or nuts should be avoided by infants until ages 1, 2, or 3 years. The most current recommendations from the American Academy of Pediatrics say that there's no evidence to support avoiding highly allergenic foods past 4-6 months of age. Some evidence is emerging from recent trials that early introduction of highly allergenic foods may even promote tolerance, but if a baby's sibling has a peanut allergy, blood testing (IgE) before peanut introduction might be useful to provide evidence that this allergy is unlikely.

Myth: Children Outgrow Allergies

Fact: Unfortunately, although children are ten times more likely than adults to have food allergies, many children may outgrow food allergies only to develop others. Some researchers believe that as a person's gastrointestinal system develops, it gets better at blocking the absorption of components that trigger food allergies. Over time, children typically outgrow allergies to cow's milk, eggs, wheat, and soybean products. Allergies to peanuts, tree nuts, fish, and shellfish, however, are more likely to be lifelong. And some children will outgrow one allergy only to develop another.

Myth: Wearing Gloves will Protect You from Poison Ivy

Fact: "Leaves of three, let them be," runs the standard advice on how to avoid poison ivy and its equally villainous cousins, poison oak and poison sumac. But those who are allergic to this relative of the cashew—as many as 85 percent of all Americans—find that no amount of armor or vigilance can protect them. The chemical that gives these plants their poisonous reputation is an oily resin called urushiol. And what makes it truly diabolical is that it can hitchhike on clothing, dog's fur, and even garden tools. If you come into contact with poison ivy, wash the oil off (preferably with brown soap and water) within 20 to 30 minutes, before it soaks into the skin. Since the residue can remain potent for a year or more, scrub tainted items as well.

Myth: Allergies Aren't Life-Threatening

Fact: Although it rarely happens, allergies can kill. Some people have such an extreme sensitivity to a particular substance that the allergen can trigger an episode known as anaphylactic shock, a sudden, potentially fatal reaction that lowers blood pressure, swells the tongue, throat, or airways to the lungs, making it difficult to breathe. Such a reaction requires immediate medical attention. Anaphylactic shock is most often triggered by a food or drug, but it can also result from an insect sting or injections of various medical agents. People with a history of severe allergic reactions should always carry a pre-loaded syringe of epinephrine (adrenaline), which can be administered in an emergency.

Myth: Many People are Allergic to Milk

Fact: When adults react adversely to milk—from cramps, gas, and diarrhea—symptoms are often mistaken for an allergic reaction, this is actually a condition known as lactose intolerance, an inherited trait caused by the body's lack of an enzyme, lactase, needed to break down lactose, the sugar in milk or milk products. In cases of lactose intolerance, adults may use supplemental lactace—e.g., Lactaid —or consume dairy products from which lactose has been removed.

True milk allergy is only common among infants but is usually outgrown in adulthood.

Myth: People who are Allergic to Shellfish are Actually Allergic to the Iodine

Fact: Some people who are allergic to seafood avoid certain skin medications and iodine-containing medical test substances because they fear an allergic reaction. But there is no connection between allergies to fish and shellfish and allergies to iodine. Allergies to fish and shellfish are caused by the protein within these meats and not to iodine, which is not an allergen. Surveys suggest that a majority of radiologists and cardiologists routinely ask patients about shellfish allergy before administering contrast media containing iodine (agents used to demonstrate pictures on X-rays). This myth seems to have originated from a 1975 study in which patients with any kind of reported allergy were twice as likely to react to contrast agents, but this has nothing to do with iodine.

Myth: Natural ("Organic") Foods are Non-Allergenic

Fact: Limiting your diet to organic food is no guarantee that you'll avoid food allergies. In fact, some of the most allergenic foods are "natural," unprocessed foods: cow's milk, eggs, peanuts, wheat, soybeans, fish, shellfish, and tree nuts. Combined, these foods account for up to 90 percent of all ingested allergic reactions. Allergies are caused not by chemicals related to growing the food, but by proteins in the food itself.

Myth: Allergy Shots Don't Work

Fact: While immunotherapy given by injections may not work for all allergies and all people, it has been shown to be effective for allergies to insect venom 98 percent of the time, and for hay fever about 85 percent of the time. In some cases, immunotherapy can actually trigger an acute allergic reaction, but if the therapy is properly administered, these risks are minimal.

Myth: Artificial Dye can be a Common Source of Allergy

Fact: Despite controversy surrounding artificial food coloring since the 1950s, and around food additives in the 1970s, there is no scientific evidence to support a link between exposure to artificial dye or coloring and allergic reactions. Rare cases of anaphylaxis (life-threatening reactions) have been reported in reaction to carmine, a natural red coloring derived from dried insects that is commonly used in cosmetics, but not in reaction to artificial dye.

Myth: Egg in Vaccines is a Frequent Cause of Allergy

Fact: The common MMR vaccine (measles, mumps and pertussis) is safe for anyone with a history of egg allergy, with no testing or allergy referral required. Influenza vaccine also generally can be given safely to egg-allergic patients, as concluded from dozens of trials. In this latter case, the Joint Council of Allergy, Asthma, and Immunology says there's no need for a waiting period or referral to an allergy specialist, while the Centers for Disease Control and Prevention and the American Academy of Pediatrics recommend 30 minutes of observation for egg- allergic patients who receive influenza vaccine and referral to an allergist if there's a history of anaphylaxis to egg. Egg-free influenza vaccine is a relatively new alternative.

Vaccine for yellow fever or rabies is contraindicated in patients with allergy to egg, but there are tests and procedures that may allow administration of these vaccinations in a graded manner in some patients. Egg-free versions of rabies vaccine also are an alternative. Gelatin in both of these vaccines can cause allergic reactions, so one must identify gelatin-hypersensitive patients before vaccinating.

Myth: Moving to The Southwestern States will Cure Allergies

Fact: For allergy sufferers, there is simply no safe haven. While desert regions have no maple trees or ragweed, they do have plenty of other plants that produce pollen, including sagebrush and cottonwood, ash, and olive trees. Relocating to such a region may offer relief for a few months, but a fresh crop of allergies to local plants is likely to develop before long.

Myth: Penicillin Allergy is Common

Fact: Adverse reactions to antibiotics are very common, but true allergic reactions are uncommon. Approximately 10% of people in general say they are allergic to penicillin, but fewer than 10% of those will have a positive skin test or symptoms if challenged. Labeling someone allergic to this antibiotic makes them more likely to receive less-effective, more-toxic, costlier antibiotic alternatives. Thus efforts should be made to clear patients from retaining this label, if falsely applied.

Myth: Gluten is a Common Source of Allergy

Fact: Eating gluten is currently being blamed for many ills of humanity, largely driven by companies with products to sell—so you should avoid self-diagnosing a gluten allergy. True hypersensitivity reactions can occur toward wheat, rye, or barley, but generally not to gluten. Celiac disease is an autoimmune condition (not traditional hypersensitivity) that improves with a gluten-free diet. Allergic type hypersensitivity to gluten is rare, but patients more commonly report having "gluten sensitivity" and intestinal symptoms after eating foods with gluten. That's a poorly defined condition that's hard to prove. We have discussed this in chapter 39.

Myth: Mold is a Common Source Of Allergy

Fact: Mold is everywhere and can cause real problems in susceptible persons, but rarely unless ingested in large quantities. Most health problems attributed to mold exposure are exaggerated, with no scientific basis or supportive evidence. But "hysteria" around mold has been a boon to some lawyers and companies that sell air purifiers and other detoxification equipment. So don't get caught up in this hysteria.

This is a compilation of the most common myths about allergy. Hopefully this can provide you with some reassurance.

CHAPTER 48

Rapidity Of Weight Loss and Long Term Success: Another Myth Destroyed?

Conventional wisdom dictates that gradual weight reduction for the treatment of obesity is more apt to be sustained in the long run when compared with rapid weight loss through "crash diets" of any type. I had always subscribed to this former notion until it was subjected to objective research—invariably a good idea that often debunks so-called "common sense."

The following study to which I refer should form the basis of future research for confirmation; that's how science works.

The study[63] was a two-phase randomized trial in a Melbourne (Australia) metropolitan hospital. It included 204 volunteers (51 men and 153 women) aged 18 to 70 years, who were quite obese (body mass index between 30 and 45) During phase 1, they randomly assigned the subjects to enter a 12-week rapid weight loss program, or a 36-week gradual program, both aimed at a 15% weight loss. Those participants who lost 12.5% or more of their body weight during phase 1 went on a weight maintenance diet for 144 weeks (phase 2). The primary outcome was the residual weights of both groups at the end of the study (week 144).

Of the 200 participants, half were randomly assigned to the gradual weight loss group and the remaining half, the rapid weight loss group. After phase 1, 50% of the participants in the gradual weight loss group, and 81% in the rapid weight loss group achieved 12·5% or more weight loss in their allocated times, and these latter participants who had lost this weight then entered into phase 2. At the end of this latter phase, although both gradual weight loss and rapid weight loss participants had regained most of their lost weight, there was no significant difference between the two groups (gradual weight loss regained 71·2% of their lost weight, versus rapid weight loss, 70·5%).

From these data the authors concluded: "The rate of weight loss does not affect the proportion of weight regained within 144 weeks. These findings are not consistent with present dietary guidelines which recommend gradual over rapid weight loss, based on the belief that rapid weight loss is more quickly regained."

But their conclusion, while correct, requires some qualification. First, a greater proportion of individuals in the rapid weight loss program achieved an initial significant weight reduction, as opposed to those in the gradual category. Second, most of the initial weight reduction was regained at the later—longer—interval in both groups. This finding is consistent with our long-held belief that those who are obese have great difficultly maintaining a satisfactory weight in the long run—no matter how they initially reduce. This, unfortunately, is the sad truth.

Conclusion:

Even though the odds for long-term success are stacked against those who are obese, they should initially try to get the weight off as promptly as possible through any possible safe program. Then work like a demon to keep it off afterwards through whatever means one can conjure up, but—let's face it—basic and permanent lifestyle changes will also be necessary. Personally, I have yet to find the "holy grail."

C✒CHAPTER 49✒⁀

Commercial Air Travel: How Safe is it?

Because of an unusual number of air crashes that occur periodically, many of us are tempted to conclude that such travel is unsafe. But is it really? Despite widespread media coverage of each tragic event, the actual numbers continue to indicate that air travel remains quite safe, amounting to 0.019 fatalities per 100 million individual miles traveled. To gain perspective, compare that rate with automobile travel, which claims approximately 1.13 fatalities per 100 million vehicle miles traveled, which is a rate 60 times higher than air travel.

A bigger danger in air travel—although still quite low—lies within the cabin itself. Because an aircraft cabin is an enclosed space, passengers are exposed to infectious agents expelled by sneezes or coughs from sick passengers. Nevertheless, research suggests the air on a plane is generally not a cause for great worry. More important, however, is who sits near you. Most commercial flights use recirculated air as opposed to fresh air from outside the plane. Fresh air may sound cleaner, but 50 percent or more of recirculated air travels through high-efficiency filters that eliminate 97 to 99 percent of the bacteria, viruses, fungi and dust. Also, most aircraft circulates air side-to-side in sections of the plane, rather than the length of the cabin, limiting exposure to airborne particles.

A study in the *Journal of the American Medical Association*[64] disclosed that, on flights from San Francisco to Denver, passengers in airplanes with recirculated air reported no more colds or other infections than passengers in planes using fresh air. Your proximity to someone with a cold or flu, however, does seem to matter. A review of research in the medical journal *Lancet*[65] concluded that the risk of becoming newly infected while airborne—during a flight of eight hours or more—is most closely associated with sitting within two rows of an already-infected person.

The overall risk is similar to the risk in other confined spaces such as a bus, train, or classroom. Just as in those circumstances, on an airplane you may not always be able to avoid being close to someone who is coughing and sneezing. But good hygiene can help prevent infections. This includes washing your hands before eating and not touching your nose, eyes, or mouth during the flight. If you currently have a cold or other upper respiratory infection, try to avoid public travel, but if that's impossible, I suggest wearing a facemask (N-95 respirator mask). The same type of mask can be used for those sitting near an infected passenger or for those having any conditions that can reduce resistance to airborne infections.

Another cause of concern has arisen from a recent study, in which Auburn University researchers, in a study presented at the 114th General Meeting of the American Society for Microbiology (2014), found that illness-causing bacteria can linger on airplane surfaces for up to a week. This group took samples from six materials, including armrests, tray tables, and seating material—upon which they applied antibiotic resistant bacteria. Then they exposed the materials to typical airplane conditions. The bacteria survived for up to a week on some surfaces, especially the seatback pockets and armrests. In order to prevent illnesses from these sources, precautions again include using alcohol wipes or a hand sanitizer when you fly, and avoid touching your nose, mouth, and eyes.

Conclusion:

Despite what you may think, flying is really quite safe, but take a few precautions as noted above.

CHAPTER 50

The Polygraph ("Lie Detector") Test: Itself The Biggest Lie?

Recently I came across one of television's true historical crime programs that presented a provocative example: A women had been brutally murdered in her apartment. During the subsequent investigation, her former boyfriend with whom she had recently had a vigorous altercation became the leading murder suspect. During the investigation, this man was "asked" to undergo a polygraph (lie detector) test in the attempt to establish his likely guilt or innocence. He agreed to be tested and was found to have "failed," thus presumably establishing his likely guilt. Despite this result, however, the evidence presented at the trial was deemed insufficient for a guilty verdict, and he was acquitted. Convinced that the polygraph test was accurate, however, his entire local community rendered him a pariah; he was shunned and even threatened with bodily harm. Several months later, however, another man, the actual murderer, was apprehended and convicted. Thus for this earlier suspect, despite his ordeal, the story had a satisfactory ending.

Conclusion:

The lie detector test itself was inaccurate and misleading!

As a result, this case provoked in me serious questions that should be amenable to modern scientific evaluation, namely, what do these polygraph tests consist of, and how often are they inaccurate? Interestingly, the challenge presented by this case is strikingly similar to those we face regularly as medical practitioners when we evaluate various tests in the attempt to establish the presence of many diseases. For this reason, I present the results of my investigation below:

Consistent with my experience cited above, the American public seems to be convinced that the "lie detector" is valid, as indicated by its ubiquitous use in "whodunit" literature, and on television crime, psychology, talk, and news shows. After all, faced with such an avalanche of widespread approbation, who could doubt the validity of such a test? Supporting this illusion is the fact that state and local police departments and law enforcement agencies across the United States are generally avid proponents of this method. But let's take a critical look at this subject.

The Procedure and its History

This test has been used for nearly a century, and it employs a "polygraph," which, during questioning, continuously records an examinee's blood pressure, respiration, pulse rate, and skin resistance (an indirect measure of perspiration).

The usual format compares responses to "relevant" questions" with those of "control" questions. The control questions are designed to control for the effect of the generally threatening nature of relevant questions. Control questions concern misdeeds that are similar to those being investigated, but refer to the subject's past and are usually broad in scope; for example, "Have you ever betrayed anyone who trusted you?"

A person who is telling the truth is assumed to fear control questions more than relevant questions. This is because control questions are designed to arouse a subject's concern about their past truthfulness, while relevant questions ask about a crime of which they are suspected. A pattern of greater physiological response to relevant questions than to control questions leads to a diagnosis of "deception." Greater response to control questions leads to a judgment of no deception. If no difference is found between relevant and control questions, the test result is considered "inconclusive."

The test records the activity of the sympathetic branch of the autonomic (involuntary) nervous system that influences heart rate, respiratory rate, blood pressure, and perspiration. Although this part of the nervous system is active at all times, it increases during excitement, rage, anxiety, fear or fright, any of which could be caused by lying. But deception is a cognitive function that defies direct measurement. Indeed, throughout the entire history of medical science, there have been no scientific studies that have shown that the emotional response linked to lying could be measured. Moreover, reactions associated with lying and any other assumed emotional stresses can be quite variable. Some people may stay calm with a gun at their head. By contrast, others may respond excessively with heart thumping and sweaty palms at simply shaking someone's hand. And the polygraph examination itself often causes fear and anxiety, and if such responses are excessive in response to a given question, then one may be deemed to have failed that question by a polygraph examiner.

The Evidence

Because of this obvious biologic improbability in this era of evidence-based medical science, the premise of lie detection by polygraph has fallen under a cloud of skepticism, justly considered as pseudoscience by most of the scientific community[66]

The American Polygraph Association (APA) is a professional organization for polygraph examiners that has complete faith in the accuracy of the test. They have licensing procedures in 28 states and their own trade journal *Polygraph* in which they report scientifically questionable studies and provide anecdotes of the accuracy of their trade. The majority of these members complete a 6 week to 6 month post-high school training course in the art of polygraphy. They have no formal training in medicine, psychology, physiology, or behavior; the very disciplines on which the testing is based. The majority of their members cater to the legal system upon which their economic livelihood depends, thus creating the background for a clear conflict of interest.

As expected, polygraph examiners will usually and confidently state that the exam is highly accurate, in the neighborhood of a 95%. This implies that if 100 guilty suspects are given a polygraph exam, 95 of them will be detected through the test, meaning that only five of these 100 will be a false negative and not be detected by this method. On the other hand, they will state that if you are telling the truth then you have almost a 100% chance of being cleared by the test[67].

But in order to pass muster with modern science, the two characteristics that must be established are the *sensitivity* and *specificity* of this test: Sensitivity is that percentage of positive test results when lying is known to exist. Specificity is the percentage of negative results in the absence of prevarication. Under both scenarios, in order to establish the test's accuracy, the presence of both lying and honesty must be known prior to—and independent of—the test procedure itself. True accuracy must be derived from real-life conditions because, for obvious reasons, it cannot be derived from volunteers in laboratory settings that lack the emotional pressures of real suspicion. In order to accomplish this, a group without known prevarication is tested to assess the results. But absolute proof of honesty is evasive in such individuals, because even if lying is absent, the anxiety associated with the test may cause false positive test results, reducing test specificity, and this appears to be a major confounder.

Even more problematic, however, is the testing of subjects who are proven to be guilty. Such guilty subjects—and many others—can purposely control their reactions (termed "countermeasures"), sufficiently to confuse the results enough to produce a "false negative." One outstanding example of a false negative was that of Aldrich Ames, who, in 1995, had successfully passed five polygraphs during his long career in intelligence, and, despite this, he was subsequently arrested and convicted of spying. In 2003 another example was provided by Gary Ridgway, who eventually was found to be the Green River Killer, having murdered 49 women in the Seattle area. Ironically, Ridgway had passed a lie detector test in 1987, while another man—who was proved to be innocent—failed.

Also impugning the accuracy of this test is the fact that establishing true "guilt" often results from use of prior polygraphic testing which may contribute to confessions and/or guilty verdicts in court, skewing the data toward a falsely high accuracy (sensitivity) of the test. Under most circumstances, the testing examiner also usually has prior suspicions about the honesty of the examinee, and this can cause bias in the test's interpretation. Establishing true sensitivity of this test, therefore, is unlikely ever to be achieved. I am also told by police representatives that the skill of the examiner also creates marked variability of results, creating a major source of inaccuracy.

Some smaller police departments with limited budgets may designate a police officer to be their department examiner instead of using an outside professional examiner. The designated testing officer may have little or no formal training, other than the limited training provided by the company selling the instrument to the police department.

Police officers conducting polygraph examinations can lead to situational bias based upon an officer's predisposition to believe most suspects are generally guilty, and as a result, if a response is inconclusive the officer may categorize it as untruthful.

If the officer conducting the test is aware of the circumstances of the individual being tested, and the weight and extent of the evidence indicating the individual being tested is the perpetrator of the crime, unbiased testing is virtually impossible.

Officers are also generally trained to ask questions using phrasing that may cause someone to answer in a manner that may appear to be an admission of guilt. This type of questioning format would be inappropriate in a polygraph examination.

Critical and Scientific Study

The polygraph was not subjected to modern critical and scientific investigation until the past three decades[68,69]. Since then there have been several studies employing improved methodology which, despite the impossibility of achieving a completely satisfactory research design, clearly refute the high accuracy previously claimed. These studies have appeared in reputable peer-reviewed journals[70]. They generally report a sensitivity ranging around 76 percent and a specificity of 52 percent. This means that out of 100 liars only 76 of them will be detected by the polygraph. But what is even more astonishing is the specificity of 52 percent, meaning that out of 100 people who are not lying, only 52 will be identified as telling the truth while 48 of these honest individuals will be branded as liars. These odds are similar a coin toss which would have a specificity of 50 percent. Other studies[71,72,73] have shown even lower levels of accuracy, casting doubt upon the rationale of using this test for any purpose whatsoever.

In 2003, the National Academy of Sciences (NAS), after a comprehensive review, issued a report entitled "The Polygraph and Lie Detection," stating that the majority of polygraph research was "unreliable, unscientific and biased", concluding that 57 of approximately 80 research studies— upon which the American Polygraph Association relies—were significantly flawed. It concluded that, although the test performed better than chance in catching lies—far from perfect—perhaps most importantly, they found the test produced too many false positives.

If anything, there is perhaps one minor advantage to subjecting suspected felons to such testing[74,75] for 25 to 50 percent of examinees will, under the intense psychological pressure of the exam, confess to the misdeed at hand, having been persuaded that they have been proven dishonest by "scientific" means. It is usual for the polygraph examiners to interrogate the subjects who have "failed" the test. Examiners may state that there is no way now to deny the objective guilt demonstrated by this "impartial" scientific device, and that the only available option is to confess, which they often do. But, while perhaps effective, this in no way exonerates the test itself. Perhaps various forms of torture such as water boarding might be just as effective. And one might ask further how often this form of interrogation might lead innocent persons to falsely admit, out of fear or other threats, to some form of wrongdoing.

Justification for Continued Use?

For the reasons stated above, the continued use of polygraphic lie detection has the potential to cause much harm to those many innocents who are falsely judged dishonest by its results. A single failure could conceivably ruin one's life. Since 1923, polygraph evidence has not been admissible in federal court cases because the test was deemed to lack scientific validity. Sadly, however, it is still used widely by the court systems of many states. Moreover, suspects are frequently "offered" this test prior to criminal proceedings, but if, for any reason, they decline to be tested, this refusal alone may cause them to be presumed guilty. Conversely, if they consent to be tested, they are risking the commonly occurring false positive outcome, which in the view of prosecutors and juries, supports a guilty verdict. Thus from the standpoint of the accused, he/she is caught in a "catch 22" situation.

Even more regrettable is the attempted application of this testing for pre-employment or security clearance. In this context, testing large groups that are predominantly honest will disclose a large number of false positive responses, as encompassed in the mathematical principles of Bayes theorem[76]. Understanding these concepts, the American Medical Association's Council on Scientific Affairs (1986) has recommended that the polygraph not be used in pre-employment screening and security clearance, with which I fully concur.

Adding clear restrictions to this testing, The Federal Employee Polygraph Protection Act, passed in 1988, virtually outlawed using lie detectors in connection with employment. That law covers all private employers in interstate commerce, which includes almost every private company that uses a computer, the U.S. mail, or a telephone system to send messages to someone in another state.

Under the Act, it is illegal for all private companies to:

1.   Require, request, suggest, or cause any employee or job applicant to submit to a lie detector test.

2.   Use, accept, refer to, or inquire about the results of any lie detector test conducted on an employee or job applicant.

3.   Dismiss, discipline, discriminate against, or even threaten to take action against any employee or job applicant who refuses to take a lie detector test.

The law also prohibits employers from discriminating against or firing those who claim its protections.

Federal applicants and employees are also generally protected from lie detector tests by civil service rules. Despite all these apparent safeguards, they often must submit to a polygraph examination in the quest of coveted security clearance for federal employment, or to retain such a job. The Employee Polygraph Protection Act allows polygraph tests to be used in connection with jobs in security and handling drugs, or in investigating a specific theft or other suspected crimes.

Defying reason, these examinations are used by agencies such as the FBI, CIA, and National Security Agency where they are commonplace. Applicants might expect them even before they start working at the agency. They may also be required to take follow-up polygraph tests from time to time to time. But the first polygraph occurs at the initial screening. That often happens when, prior to a likely job offer, the only thing left is the polygraph test. The need to pass can be a very nervous event for anyone—especially those who have not been subjected to a polygraph before, and of course, as explained, this can easily trigger a false positive response, resulting in an unjustified rejection. Thus use of such a test for this purpose is very difficult to defend.

Conclusion:

Finally, in summarizing its many pitfalls in 2001, Iacono[77] stated in an article entitled Forensic Lie Detection: Procedures without Scientific Basis, the following: "Although this form of testing may be useful as an investigative aid and tool to induce confessions, it does not pass muster as a scientifically credible test. Its theory is based on naive, implausible assumptions indicating

1.   That it is biased against innocent individuals.

2.   That it can be beaten simply by artificially augmenting responses to control questions. Although it is not possible to adequately assess the error rate of this test, both of these conclusions are supported by published research findings in the best social science journals.

It is time to ban polygraphic testing across the board. Any remaining state or federal laws that allow use of the polygraph, in or outside of court settings, must be abolished.

Unfortunately, however, various state and national polygraph certifying and licensing organizations—whose livelihood depends upon their own continued existence—are well entrenched in our society. Their provision of services to most law enforcement agencies creates a symbiotic relationship that is difficult to overcome. As a result, correcting this problem, unfortunately, is likely to remain intractable. Nevertheless, in order to eradicate this blight, it is incumbent on the scientific community, as well as others who understand these concepts, to educate the public about this perversion of science and relentlessly urge the responsible authorities to discontinue the present unsatisfactory status quo.

CHAPTER 51

Stretching before Exercise: Another Myth

Almost all of us see—or participate personally in—static stretching before engaging in strenuous exercise of most types. By stretching, I mean slowly moving muscles until they just start to hurt and then holding the stretch briefly. The reasons for stretching are presumably to reduce the chances for injury and to increase performance. Although we in medicine have long recognized that little scientific evidence supports these assumptions, recent evidence indicates that stretching not only fails to prevent injuries, but actually impairs strength and speed in some athletes. Thus stretching should be limited or excluded before most physical activity.

One recent study, published in the *Journal of Strength and Conditioning Research*[78], concluded that if you stretch before you lift weights, you may actually feel weaker and wobblier than you would have otherwise experienced. This added to accumulating prior data that support a scientific consensus that stretching is not only useless but actually likely counterproductive.

With regard to exercises of strength, e.g., weightlifting, reviews of multiple past studies have shown that prior stretching actually reduced lifting power by as much as 5-8%

when those who stretched were compared with those who didn't.

This information merely confirms what most physical trainers have already long put into practice. Most suggest just a little light and brief stretch beforehand, and spending more time on recovery stretching afterwards. This group has long felt that the best time to stretch is after exercise, but even this assumption lacks a sound scientific basis.

So stretching has long occupied an indelible part of the pre-workout routine for misguided reasons: Although it seems to help in a limited degree with flexibility and improve range of motion, many falsely equate stretching with the warming up of muscles. This latter activity is useful and well established. For example, tennis players require a few minutes of prior motions of various strokes, and relief pitchers need a few minutes in the bull pen before entering a game. Thus the warm-up phenomenon is well established in virtually all sports in order to enhance initial performance. But there is little evidence that either warming up or stretching prevents injuries. In contrast to warming up, stretching is potentially harmful to muscles because they may actually lose flexibility when they are overworked, and this can lead to reduction of power.

But stretching isn't all bad, for it can give non-competitive people a wider range of motion in their joints, which can help them to perform their daily activities and improve balance and posture, which can aid in preventing falls and other injuries as people age. But, as noted, the risks of stretching include decreased strength, especially in weight-bearing activities. Those who are recovering from injuries, in which there may be considerable scar tissue that limits range of motion, may also require a bit more stretching to prevent further damage to the areas involved.

So, in summary, when it comes to preparing for a workout, one should consider warming up the body rather than simply stretching muscles. That means adding exercises in addition to light stretching, like motions simulating the imminent activity, which can prepare the body for intensive motion without making the muscles vulnerable to overwork.

CHAPTER 52

Medical Tests and Yearly Checkups: Are They Really Necessary?

G eneral health check-ups have long been popular in the US, where they are often carried out yearly. By contrast, they have only recently been introduced in the UK, but to be done every five years, and this latter check-up is mainly focused on reducing the risk of heart and circulatory diseases. Doctors measure blood pressure, cholesterol levels, and body mass index and give some general health advice. If any abnormalities are found, then follow-up evaluations and/or treatment should be done at the advice of the physician.

Having a regular yearly check-up for someone who is basically healthy sounds like common sense—the ultimate in preventative medicine—but this is surprisingly controversial. That's because this is a form of screening—in other words, looking for illness in people who have no symptoms. And screening has a nasty habit of doing more harm than good, especially in the absence of evidence to prove its worth in reducing disease and mortality. The most recent trial,[79] and one of the largest ever, looked at nearly 60,000 Danish people who were offered annual checks for five years. Five years after this period, there was no effect on heart attacks or overall death rates.

The potential downside of screening is that it can worry people unnecessarily, offer false reassurance, or trigger unneeded tests and treatments. That has been shown for certain kinds of screening (see below).

Female Examinations

Now routine pelvic (vaginal) exams for women are meeting the same skepticism. A recent study published in a leading internal medicine journal[80] has arrived at the conclusion that this type of examination should be dropped from routine care—if it is performed on symptom-free women who are not pregnant. The study was based on a review that found no studies supporting the pelvic exam for finding ovarian cancer or any other serious disease. Exceptions to this recommendation are the periodic obtaining of so-called "PAP smears," i.e. sampling of cells from the uterine cervix to detect early cancer, but this test can be done every three years. Of course if any woman has any symptoms pointing toward this area, such as pelvic pain, abnormal bleeding, sexual dysfunction, or other troubling complaints, more frequent examinations are usually needed.

Childhood Evaluations

One need for regular yearly evaluations applies to the young, for routine health visits are essential for infants, children, and adolescents. During yearly sessions, youths can receive immunizations, developmental evaluation, blood testing, and this can further allow parents to be instructed about a variety of issues surrounding child development and care.

Colonoscopy

This worthwhile procedure is capable of detecting, preventing, and curing colon cancer. In most individuals not at high risk for such cancers, colonoscopy should begin at age 50 and repeated periodically at intervals advised by the physician performing the test. In general, repeated testing is done every five years until the age of 75. If no cancer or precancerous polyps are found initially, however, one can usually wait for 10 years for the next test. After age 75, testing usually is discontinued. For adults over 75 who have not previously been screened, decisions about first-time screening is usually made in the context of the individual's health status and competing risks. For persons older than 85 years, competing causes of mortality usually preclude any possible benefits, and thus this procedure is not indicated.

Mammography

For the average woman, the U.S. Preventive Services Task Force recommended (2009) mammography every two years in women between the ages of 50 and 74. The Canadian Task Force on Preventive Health Care (2012) and the European Cancer Observatory (2011) recommends mammography every 2-3 years between 50 and 69. After the age of 74, testing is optional and best done at the advice of your physician. These task force reports point out that, in addition to unnecessary surgery and anxiety, the risks of more frequent mammograms include a small but significant increase in breast cancer induced by radiation. Most studies do not find an effect of mammography screening on total cancer mortality. Thus when such information is offset by the fact that many women with "positive" mammography results will be suspected and treated unnecessarily for benign conditions and experience psychological distress including anxiety and uncertainty for years, we must conclude that universal screening is of questionable value at best.

In high risk groups, such as those with a strong family history of breast cancer, screening does make sense. In women who are otherwise healthy, screening with mammography is probably optional, but most data suggest that this is best accomplished when augmented by careful palpation of the breasts done by self-examination or by a medical professional. When both examinations detect an area of increased density, then more intensive evaluation is justified and is more likely to yield a significant reduction of long-term mortality.

PSA Testing

PSA is a blood test designed to detect early prostate cancer in men, and it too is falling under increasing scrutiny. A growing consensus suggests that it's usually not necessary, but considerable disagreement persists. My take on this subject is that men should not routinely get this test, especially if they are younger than 50 or older than 74. If, however, you are between those ages, talk with your doctor about the risks and benefits of the test, and your risk factors, such as being African-American or having a strong family history of this disease.

Lung Cancer Tests: Only For Long-Term Smokers

A recent study found that annual low-dose CT lung scans could cut the risk of death from cancer by 16%.in long-term heavy smokers. At present, Medicare refuses to cover the cost of this test, but they should. Thus the test should be employed in those between ages 55 and 80 who smoked a pack per day for 30 years or two packs for 15 years, provided that they currently smoke or stopped within the past 15 years.

Conclusion:

I might conclude by offering the following general advice: One should always designate a personal physician (usually a family physician or general internist). An initial visit should be scheduled to include a physical examination, a general blood profile that includes cholesterol and other markers for cardiovascular risk and diabetes, an electrocardiogram, and a chest X-ray. This should be followed by advice about life-style issues such as exercise, diet, and others as needed. After that, follow-up examinations can be performed on an as-needed basis, depending primarily on the initial assessment. If no abnormalities are found to warrant closer follow-up, for men, a regular five-yearly interval to measure blood pressure and focus mainly reducing risk of heart and circulatory diseases would be quite sufficient. As noted above, women should be followed in a similar fashion, but need a bit more attention, at least with regard to PAP smears at three-yearly intervals, and for those over the age of 50, mammograms every two years are probably OK, but stay tuned regarding this later recommendation. Colonoscopy, lung scans, and PSA testing have been covered above.

TRICKS

ᐸᔑ◯CHAPTER 53◯ᔑᐳ

False Cures: Don't Be a Sucker!

As of 2007, about 40% of Americans opted for questionable treatments that range from those simply unproven to those that are outright frauds. These diverse methods encompass practitioners of alternative medicine (employing herbs and dietary supplements and others), spinal manipulation, acupuncture, "energy healing," and many more. Not only are we being duped, but many states actually sanction many dubious practices. At this time, seventeen states, the District of Columbia, Puerto Rico, and the Virgin Islands license naturopaths. Forty states license acupuncturists. Chiropractors are licensed in all 50 states. The Affordable Care Act mandates coverage of "state licensed alternative medicine practitioners" including "wellness" clinics that can employ "energy" healers and herbalists.

So after over a century of painstaking rigorous scientific advances, we preserve a mishmash of unproven methods that offer dubious "cures." The U.S. Congress has fostered this situation by passing ill-advised laws that led to the establishment of what was the Office of Alternative Medicine, later named the National Center for Complementary and Alternative Medicine (NCCAM), and again renamed the National Center for Complementary and Integrative Health (NCCIH) at the National Institutes of Health. Defying modern concepts of science, since 1999 this agency has awarded over $2 billion to non-evidence-based practice schools for naturopaths, acupuncturists, chiropractors, and oriental medicine practitioners[81], meaning that even the United States government is granting de facto approval of these questionable methods. Moreover, many private insurance plans are also now covering the highly doubtful procedure of acupuncture[82], although Medicare (parts A and B) does not presently provide compensation for this method. Not only has NCCIH been awarding grants for training and career development for alternative medicine practitioners, but they are also supporting research that would presumably test whether or not these methods are beneficial. Despite such funding, however, published results for such trials are rare indeed, and whenever this does occur, the "researchers" seldom provide precise statements. The protocols are usually poorly designed, non-evidence based trials. Despite these obvious deficiencies, this U.S. agency continues to funnel taxpayer funds into dubious research on unproven—even disproven—alternative medicine protocols. One study[83] tracked $2 billion in research grants to test the success of these methods, and it yielded no positive result that would alter current evidenced-based medical practice.

In order to understand why we have been so terribly misguided, we need to examine briefly the modern criteria required to prove the benefit of any method of treatment:

First, we usually form a hypothesis based upon biologic plausibility. This depends upon fundamental knowledge of biology, which is usually supported by preliminary observations. For instance, long ago a fungus, later called penicillin, was found to be capable of killing disease-producing microbes in the laboratory. This then led to numerous trials in humans to see if various infections could respond to this antibiotic and yet be free of any toxic effect from the penicillin itself. Needless to say, the rest is history.

In most cases, repeated study from varying sites and researchers is required to confirm that a proposed new treatment is really effective. This laborious process usually involves many volunteer human subjects with a given malady that are divided into two groups—treated and untreated (control group)—to ascertain whether the new method really accounts for improvement. Ideally, neither the patients nor the dispensers of the new treatment are aware of which ones are actually receiving the new, presumably active, agent. This process is termed "double blinding." Statistical methods are used to determine the numerical validity of the resulting responses. In some cases, as in the case of surgical or manipulative procedures, blinding is not feasible, but comparison with some type of control group is usually necessary. These controls may consist of those left untreated, or those receiving competing methods. When possible, sham methods can be used as controls, as in the case of acupuncture (small pointed objects such as toothpicks are applied to non-acupuncture sites). In this latter instance, the results from the most carefully executed protocols regularly show no significant difference between those treated and the sham controls. Any study lacking double blinding is considered less robust, and in most cases, repeated research employing differing methods and study groups is necessary in order to confirm the validity of the initial results.

As noted, whenever the "alternative" medical treatments are subjected to these same rigorous standards demanded by modern science, they clearly do not work. Although NCCIH was launched with the claim that it would separate what is useful from what is not, it has not done this.

Moreover, NCCIH has never concluded that a method should be discarded as a result of testing or because it lacks a plausible rationale.

Worse yet, its funding of "complementary medicine" centers in qualified medical schools has created quackery-infested nests throughout our sanctioned and mainstream medical education system.

From this information, it is obvious that further testing of such "alternative" methods is clearly a waste of scarce research funds. This is best summarized in a comprehensive report by W.I. Sampson, MD, on the popular website, Quackwatch[84], calling for the defunding and dissolution of NCCIH. I fully concur.

CHAPTER 54

Snake Oil Rises Again—The Anatomy of a Typical Scam

New health frauds pop up continuously, but promoters usually fall back on the same old clichés and tricks to gain your trust and get your money. The following four points should serve as red flags to alert the consumer of likely fraud:

1.   The vendor or practitioner claims the treatment or product works by a secret formula. Legitimate scientists share their knowledge so their peers can review the data.

2.   The treatment is supposedly an amazing or miraculous breakthrough or cure. Real medical breakthroughs are few and far between, and when they happen, are not touted as amazing or miraculous by any responsible scientist or journalist.

3.   The treatment is publicized only in the back pages of magazines, over the phone, by direct mail, in newspaper ads pretending to be news stories, or on 30-minute, talk-show-format infomercials. The results of studies on bona fide treatments are generally reported first in peer-reviewed medical journals.

4.   Proof for the treatment relies solely on testimonials from satisfied customers. These people may never have had the disease the product is supposed to cure, may be paid representatives, or may simply not exist. Often they're identified only by initials or first names.

The following description exemplifies all these elements of a typical scam. Although it is by no means unique, it contains several important and instructive features:

It begins with a large paid advertisement in local Newspaper, bearing the title:

TV Talk Show Doctor's Shocking Revelation

The article opens by stating; "Recently, alternative medicine expert Bryce Wylde, a frequent guest on the Dr. Oz Show, revealed a simple secret that amazed millions who suffer with digestion nightmares. And people haven't stopped talking about it since." The ad goes on to identify AloeCure[R], a preparation of Aloe Vera, as this magic treatment, a substance that has been applied externally for centuries supposedly to hasten wound healing. The ad suggests that the soothing relief is transferable to the stomach, where it can "neutralize acid" and relieve everything from "gastric reflux pain (heartburn), irritable bowel syndrome, Crohn's disease, colitis, constipation and a host of other digestive problems."

But first a few words about "Doctor" Bryce Wylde: He is known as one of "Canada's leading alternative health experts," being a natural healthcare practitioner whose specialty is homeopathy, clinical nutrition, supplementation, and botanical medicine, whose focus is routed within "functional" medicine. He graduated with a B.Sc. Hons. (BioPsyc) from York University in Toronto. He went on to pursue a career in complementary alternative medicine and nutrition, graduating with a Diploma in Homeopathic

Medicine and Health Sciences (DHMHS) from the Ontario College of Homeopathic Medicine. I add parenthetically that homeopathy is largely debunked worldwide and considered by the scientific community as a form of quackery. Interestingly, his picture is shown with a stethoscope around his neck, an obvious signal to suggest the possession of authentic medical credentials.

For confirmation of the value of Aloe Vera, the ad above seeks quotations from the following "experts":

1.   Doug Jewett, CEO of American Global Health Group (AGHG), states that, "More than ever, I want to introduce digestion sufferers to our remarkable product, improve their health while saving them money, and provide long lasting relief." I discovered that this company, notwithstanding its name, lists a vice president and a single employee with an estimated annual income of $160,000.

2.   Dr. Liza Leal, an individual family physician from Texas, who, along with her office associate, Duncen G. Foulds (oral surgeon), are the authors of a self-published book entitled "LIVE WELL WITH CHRONIC PAIN." Dr. Leal has been a practicing physician for fifteen years and is currently the Director of the Medical-Dental Institute in Sugar Land. Texas. As a member of the "AGHG team," Dr. Leal is listed as "an expert in the uses of Aloe Vera for both medical and dental purposes."

3.   Dr. Santiago Rodriguez, PhD states that "Just two ounces of AloeCure reduces the acids in your stomach by ten times" Working with Global Health Group, Dr. Rodriguez supposedly functions as a research chemist "specializing in Aloe Vera" Their sales center is located at the AGHG headquarters in

Seattle, Washington, USA, with an Asian sales center in Guangdong, China, operating with three wholly owned subsidiaries: Taishan AGHG Aloe Products Co. Ltd, which operates the production facility in China; Global Health (Taishan) Plantation Co. Ltd, the operator of two farms in Taishan; and Hainan Zhengran Aloe Development Co. Ltd, operating AGHG's largest plantation base, located on Hainan Island in the middle of the South China Sea. Thus the Aloe Vera product is obviously obtained from and likely produced in China, far from being known as a sound source of pristine and unadulterated products.

4.   Francisco DeWeever, a "Certified Nutritional Microscopist," states that, "My patients report their IBS (irritable bowel syndrome), Crohn's, Colitis, Constipation, Acid-Reflux, and a host of other digestive problems have all but disappeared." DeWeever is listed as President & CEO at ReNewHealth Wellness Center St. Maarten, Dutch Caribbean. Nutritional microscopy, also known as Live Blood Analysis, is supposedly a procedure for obtaining a "quick and accurate assessment of your blood, able to provide a composite of over 25 aspects from your live blood. It allows observers to detect multiple vitamin and mineral deficiencies, toxicity, tendencies toward allergic reaction, excess fat circulation, liver weakness and arteriosclerosis." Needless to say, this technique has never been recognized as a bona fide scientific method, and never will.

And, of course, next comes a satisfied patient, a certain Ralph Burns (which one?) rounds it out by providing the usual testimonial: "I was tortured for years by my Acid Reflux. Sometimes I'd almost pass out from the pain. My wife suffers with digestion problems too. If she eats one thing wrong, she spends hours stuck in the bathroom dealing with severe bouts of constipation or diarrhea."

The ad also states that the FDA warns about popular antacids posing a risk of hip, wrist, and spine fractures. They contrast this with the claim that their own natural digestion solution poses "no possible side effects." Finally Jewett states that Major Drug Companies are threatened by their "Natural Digestion Remedy," suggesting that, out of fright, these companies may threaten to take appropriate legal action supposedly against AGHD, but he further asserts that; "we're not going to be intimidated."

Does the Product Work?

After a thorough search of the world's published scientific literature, I found ten studies that provided at least limited information about this subject[85]. In no studies was aloe vera administered internally with the intention of relieving gastrointestinal distress of any type, although in some cases, diarrhea was caused by this agent, thus relieving constipation. Even in studies of topical application of aloe vera to promote wound healing, the evidence of benefit was unclear. Since this comprehensive review, no evidence to date has surfaced to alter these conclusions, but adverse reactions reported, such as diarrhea, electrolyte (mineral) imbalance, intestinal malabsorption, weight loss, and liver damage have provided additional, and sobering, concerns. When comparing these potential adverse reactions with those of the class of antacids (Proton Pump Inhibitors, or PPIs) implicated in bone fractures, the FDA has reviewed seven published studies, six of which reported an increased risk of fractures of the hip, wrist, and spine with the use of PPIs. They go on to state that "Based on the available data, it is not clear at this time if the use of PPIs is the cause of the increased bone fractures." They further note the "Of the people who use PPIs, the greatest increased risk for these fractures was seen in those who receive high doses of these medications or use them for a year or longer." This opens an important question: Is one willing to chance a small (known) risk of bone complications versus an unknown risk of possibly even more disastrous consequences?

Conclusion:

The information contained within this advertisement is quite informative, for it follows the general pattern presented by countless other such scams. It should raise the level of general awareness to allow one to immediately recognize and reject them immediately.

CHAPTER 55

The Use of Professional Athletes as Shills to Promote Useless Products, A.K.A. "Snake Oil"

High profile professional athletes often tout automobiles, after-shave lotions, blue jeans, and other consumer products, and this seems like "business as usual." But when such athletes enter the realm of useless health products, they are flirting with measures that are not only ineffective but could pose a danger to the public. The first example is presented below:

Super Beta Prostate. Referring to this product, Joe Theismann, the former football star, says; "Throughout my career in football, I've seen some major game-changing moments. The same goes for my own life—like when I realized the reason I was going to the bathroom so much during the day and getting up in the middle of the night to go was due to my prostate! Now that was a game changer!"

What are the facts? β-sitosterol is the ingredient in this product alleged to be effective in promoting function of the prostate gland (located at the base of the bladder and often accounting for slowing urine flow). Alone and in combination with similar plant sterols, β-sitosterol reduces blood levels of cholesterol, and is sometimes used in treating elevated levels of this substance by inhibiting cholesterol absorption in the intestine. While this substance is useful in prevention and control of cardiovascular disease, one small substandard study conducted in Europe suggested that urine flow was enhanced in those taking medicinal form of this plant sterol, and thus it has been touted for benign prostatic hyperplasia (BPH) in that continent. Nevertheless, even if proven to be effective in prostate conditions (which is doubtful), this substance is widely distributed in the plant kingdom and found in such sources as pecans, avocados, pumpkin seeds, cashews, fruit, rice bran, wheat germ, corn oils, soybeans, and others. This presents one with a veritable cornucopia of nutritious and cheaper ingredients with which to fend off cardiovascular and prostate(?) conditions.

Conclusion:

I would choose a diet that includes these latter components, but not with the intent to aid in urination. Nothing more need be said.

The next example demonstrates a worthless product combined with athletic event promotion, in this case auto racing.

Hydroxycut is a brand of dietary supplements that is marketed as another aid to weight loss. Originally developed and marketed by MuscleTech Corp., now defunct, the product was sold to Iovate Health Sciences in 2003-2004 but the latter company continues to market Hydroxycut. By 2009, about 15% of Americans were taking dietary supplements for weight loss, and Hydroxycut was among the biggest sellers, with about a million units sold each year. Average cost per person—about $1.35 daily.

Iovate Health Sciences was forced by the U.S. Food and Drug Administration (FDA) in 2004 to reformulate Hydroxycut to eliminate ephedra, a dangerous component. In 2009 this agency again issued a warning to consumers to stop using Hydroxycut products, due to 23 reports of serious health problems associated with its the use, including at least one death, and users were advised to destroy any product that they may possess. The warning stated; *"Although the liver damage appears to be relatively rare, FDA believes consumers should not be exposed to unnecessary risk. Consumers who have these products are urged to stop using them."* Following the FDA warning, the manufacturer agreed to recall the products.

After the 2009 recall, Hydroxycut was again reformulated and placed back on sale, and presumably the only ingredient carried over from prior formulations was caffeine. Providing false reassurance to the consumer, Hydroxycut is sold at conventional retailers, online retailers, and through direct television marketing. Like virtually all dietary supplements, published studies demonstrating scientific evidence of its effectiveness and safety are flimsy and riddled with conflicts of interest, or lacking altogether. Compounding the farce, Hydroxycut had been promoted as being created and endorsed by doctors. Television advertisements for Hydroxycut featured a medical resident, although reporters were unable to locate him after Hydroxycut was removed from the market in 2009.

As of 2013, the primary ingredients in the product line include Lady's mantle extract, Wild olive extract, Komijn extract, Caffeine Anhydrous (1,3,7-Trimethylxanthine) supplying 200 Mg of caffeine, Wild mint extract and, in some products, Green coffee bean extract. Despite the reformulation, these substances (except for caffeine) have been poorly studied and might actually be harmful. Side effects continue to include liver failure (requiring liver transplantation in some cases), rhabdomyolysis (extensive muscle breakdown), and one death of a 19-year-old man. Another case published in 2013 reported on a patient who developed ulcerative colitis with repeated exacerbations each time after ingesting Hydroxycut Hardcore.

Providing an advertising bonanza for the Iovate company, in March 2013 racecar driver Tony Kanaan piloted the winning No. 11 Hydroxycut IndyCar at the Indianapolis 500 and was planning to use this car in 8 other events at the 2013 IndyCar Championship series.

In my opinion, these Hydroxycut events provide evidence that the FDA, although having limited success in warnings and recalls, is in need of greater power over dietary supplements. This is unlikely to occur, given so much clamor against government agencies. Unfortunately, weight-loss supplements manufacturers care far less about their products' safety and efficacy than they do about expanding and protecting their bottom lines.

Needless to say, this is another product to avoid.

Conclusion:

In the examples cited above, the consumer is tipped off by that closing disclaimer already noted, which I repeat: "These statements have not been evaluated by the US Food and Drug Administration. These products are not intended to diagnose, treat, cure or prevent any disease." This commonly appearing statement provides the closest thing to a guarantee that you're getting ripped off with a useless product.

Anatabloc The final example demonstrates professional athletes' promotions, but with the added wrinkle—political wrongdoing.

Pro golfer Fred Couples states he takes the dietary supplement Anatabloc "to help me stay on top of my game." In this instance, Star Scientific Co., the maker of Anatabloc, touts this product through the use of this and other similar testimonials by a marathon runner, an NFL tight end, and a professional tennis player. In its marketing of the product, the company vaguely states Anatabloc helps users "reduce inflammation and support a healthy metabolism."

While Star Scientific has not made any explicit claims that Anatabloc can cure diseases, it has put out at least 15 news releases since April 2010 announcing or detailing various "scientific" studies backed by the company and indicating that anatabine, the claimed active ingredient of Anatabloc, in addition to relieving muscle aches and pains, could mitigate the underlying causes of conditions such as Alzheimer's disease, multiple sclerosis, thyroiditis, and traumatic brain injuries. The reason for all that, the company says, is attributable to anatabine's "anti-inflammatory properties." But Anatabloc, like other dietary supplements already noted, is not directly regulated by the U.S. Food and Drug Administration, and therefore, poorly studied.

In my review of the world's scientific literature, I could find only one reference to a study performed in humans, and it concluded as follows: "Anatabine supplementation had no effect on the recovery of muscle strength, hanging joint angle, arm swelling, or subjective pain ratings after a bout of maximal eccentric exercise in the forearm flexors. Therefore, it may not be beneficial for those seeking to improve recovery from heavy eccentric exercise." Interestingly, this study was funded by a research grant from Rock Creek Pharmaceuticals, Inc, a subsidiary of Star Scientific Co. I'm surprised that they allowed the manuscript to be published.

So, while the acceptance of payment by athletes and other high-profile luminaries constitutes shameful behavior, it is not illegal. Moreover, after being filmed beside a bottle of said nostrum, those shills have probably never gone near this product, and likely never will, for why should they? After all, its efficacy is supported by no credible evidence and, as usual for these and other similar products; long-term safety is seldom well monitored and always in question.

But what does this have to do with politics? Plenty! This brings us to the story of Robert McDonnell, Governor of Virginia and his wife Maureen, whose misconduct was subsequently exposed. The sordid story began with relatively trivial, if astonishingly morally obtuse, bits of graft and back-scratching. I won't bore you with the convoluted details, but will provide a brief overview:

Jonnie R. Williams Sr., CEO of Star Scientific, maker of Anatabloc, provided $15,000 to help cover the catering bill at the McDonnells' daughter's wedding — an event that took place three days after Virginia first lady Maureen McDonnell flew to Florida, where she touted Anatabloc. Among the various "goodies," monies were provided to purchase a $6,500 Rolex, complete with engraved inscription, "71st Governor of Virginia," that Williams bought for the governor at Maureen McDonnell's behest, and a $15,000 spree at Bergdorf Goodman, again on Williams' tab. Even more outrageously, Williams gave $70,000—supposedly a loan—to a corporation owned by McDonnell and his sister; plus $50,000 to Maureen McDonnell in 2011, and $10,000 as a wedding present to another McDonnell daughter.

All these gratuities were provided seemingly in exchange for the first family's ongoing touting of Anatabloc. That would represent—in anyone's book—at least a classic example of a conflict of interest, if not worse.

So, as the old saying goes, Gov. McDonnell got his hand caught in the cookie jar, but in this case it was the "snake oil jar." In this case justice was served by a court case with guilty verdict of both McDonnells. Although this verdict was subsequently reversed by the Supreme Court, it is still under study. After seeing these facts, however, what is your verdict?

CHAPTER 56

More about Dietary Supplements: Seldom Indicated and Potentially Dangerous

More than 100 million Americans consume "dietary supplements" consisting of herbal ingredients, amino acids, minerals, vitamins, and other "naturally" occurring substances. Of the huge number of unproven remedies on which about $32 billion are spent yearly, most are obtainable without a prescription from health food stores, many pharmacies, and through the Internet. Most products fall into the category of "herbal" medicines. Since they are usually considered to be "natural," most folks believe they are generally safe, which is far from the truth. In the present era, nearly 1 in 5 adults in the United States reports taking such a product, believing—without scientific evidence—that it will help them lose weight, build muscle, improve sexual virility, or fight off a variety of illnesses. The resulting products usually contain multiple substances of various chemical types. Since any given herb contains several ingredients, some manufacturers try to create standardized herbal products by identifying a suspected active ingredient and altering the manufacturing process to obtain a consistent amount of this chemical, but such attempts themselves are fraught with uncertainty created by variations in the analytical methods. For most herbs, the exact chemical, or combination of chemicals, that produces a biological effect is unknown, and it is therefore difficult—if not impossible—to create a precise "chemical fingerprint" of the herbal product. Raising the risks even further, some products are spiked illegally with hidden pharmaceuticals that may pose significant health risks, as discussed below.

The Dangers of Supplements

Here are a few hazards that I've gleaned from multiple sources, including reports of serious adverse events submitted to the U.S. Food and Drug Administration (F.D.A).

More than 6,300 adverse events associated with dietary supplements, including vitamins and herbs, were reported to the FDA from supplement companies, consumers, health-care providers, and others between 2007 and mid-April of 2012. The reports by themselves don't prove the supplements caused the problems, but these sheer numbers are cause for major concern. Symptoms range from signs of heart, kidney, or liver problems, aches, allergic reactions, fatigue, nausea, pains, and vomiting.

The reports described more than 10,300 serious outcomes (some included more than one), including 115 deaths and more than 2,100 hospitalizations, 1,000 serious injuries or illnesses, 900 emergency-room visits, and some 4,000 other important medical events.

Although the FDA gets more reports about serious problems with prescription medications than about supplements, there's a big difference between the two. That is, prescription medications may possess powerful side effects, but when used appropriately, they combat illnesses and actually save lives. By contrast, when healthy consumers use supplements, there's virtually no lifesaving effect whatsoever.

The FDA suspects most supplement problems never come to its attention, but when they do they can alert us about a developing problem. For instance, recently the agency noted seven reports of serious health problems in consumers who took Soladek vitamin solution, marketed by Indo Pharma of the Dominican Republic. When the FDA learned that tested samples contained vitamins A and D at concentrations many times the recommended daily allowances, it issued a consumer warning.

Unfortunately, current laws prevent the FDA from simply removing many suspicious products from the market. To date it has banned only one ingredient, ephedrine alkaloids. That effort dragged on for a decade, during which ephedra weight-loss products were implicated in thousands of adverse events, including deaths.

Various so-called "supplements" sold in the U.S. before 1994 were allowed to be marketed without any evidence of efficacy or safety. In 1994, after much political debate, The Dietary Supplement Health and Education Act (DSHEA) of 1994 classified "dietary supplements" as "anything" that supplements the diet—a nebulous concept indeed. This act actually worsened the situation by increasing the amount of misinformation that can be directly transmitted to prospective customers. It expanded the types of products that could be marketed as "supplements." The most logical definition of "dietary supplement" would be something that supplies one or more essential nutrients missing from the diet. DSHEA went far beyond this to include vitamins; minerals; herbs or other botanicals; amino acids; other dietary substances to supplement the diet by increasing dietary intake; and any concentrate, metabolite, constituent, extract, or combination of any such ingredients. Although many such products (particularly herbs) are marketed for their alleged preventive or therapeutic effects, the 1994 law has made it difficult or impossible for the FDA to regulate them as drugs. Since its passage, even hormones, such as melatonin, are being hawked as supplements.

The FDA has received notification of only 170 new supplement ingredients since 1994, despite an estimated 55,000 new products appearing on the market. Moreover, the F.D.A. estimates that 70% of dietary supplement companies are not regularly following basic quality control standards that would help prevent adulteration of their products. Thus only 170 (about 0.3%) of these 55,000 new supplements been studied closely enough to determine their likely side effects.

Because of these obvious shortcomings, the FDA proposed in 2011 guidance clarifying evidence necessary to assess the safety of ingredients introduced after 1994. This involved documented history of use, formulation and proposed daily dose, and duration of consumption relative to historical standards. If a new ingredient was marketed in doses exceeding those historically used, or if formulated or synthesized in a new manner, the FDA would require animal and/or historical documentation for safety. These apparently more stringent regulations remain seriously flawed, e.g., the FDA would not require studies in humans for ingredients lacking evidence of historical use. Even prior use is relevant only if one would have expected to detect adverse effects, which has seldom been accomplished in careful analyses. Even more damning, however, the new guidance would not mandate that all data—both favorable an unfavorable—be submitted to the FDA; a manufacturer could perform multiple studies and submit only the favorable data.

Thus these new guidelines would provide little assurance to the public that many of these products were actually safe. From this information, we can conclude that, unless compelling evidence indicates that any of these supplements is effective for any disorder—which is seldom the case—one should avoid all of them.

Now what's even worse is that felons are entering the mix and contaminating products with potentially toxic—and even life threatening—ingredients. On December 20, 2013, the newspaper U.S.A Today reported that numerous dietary supplement companies have been caught with adding illegal contaminants, and they are often found to be run by people with criminal backgrounds and regulatory infractions. But whether or not there is underlying criminal intent, just over half of all drug recalls in the USA from 2004 to 2012 were spiked with hidden ingredients (often drugs), according to research published in the scientific journal JAMA Internal Medicine[86]. They noted that of the 237 supplements recalled for hidden contaminants, 40% were sold for sexual enhancement, 31% for bodybuilding and 27% for weight reduction. The New York Times (Dec 22, 2013) has also weighed into this subject of toxic effects, citing that dietary supplements probably account for nearly 20% of drug-related liver injuries that require hospitalization, often leading to liver failure, the need for liver transplantation, and even death.

But don't expect the major drugstore and retail giants to provide any assurance of the quality of the products they purvey. In January, 2015, the New York State Attorney General's office accused four major retailers of selling fraudulent and potentially dangerous herbal supplements and demanded that they remove the products from their shelves. The authorities conducted tests on top-selling brands of herbal supplements at four national retailers—GNC, Target, Walgreens and Wal-Mart—and found that four out of five of the products tested did not contain any of the substances on their labels. The tests showed that pills labeled medicinal herbs often contained little more than cheap fillers like powdered rice, asparagus, and houseplants, and in some cases substances that could be dangerous to those with allergies. Following this revelation, the accused companies responded in differing ways. Most responsibly, Walgreens said it would remove the products from its shelves nationwide, even though only New York State had demanded it. Wal-Mart said it would reach out to the suppliers of its supplements "and take appropriate action." GNC said that the company would cooperate with the attorney general "in all appropriate ways," but stated less than candidly that it "stood behind the quality and purity of its store brand supplements." But before we jump to chastise these retailers for deception, it's really the entire system that lacks the necessary oversight from the ground up, and this stems from inadequate regulation by the federal government, as we note below.

Supposedly, The F.D.A. requires that companies verify that every supplement they manufacture is safe and accurately labeled. But the system essentially operates on the honor code, or perhaps the (dis)honor code? Unfortunately, dangerous supplements can easily reach the market because they are not subject to a review or approval process. Under current law, supplements are assumed to be safe until the authorities can prove otherwise. And in general, they are pulled from shelves only after serious injuries occur, which is not uncommon. Now we have evidence that a State (New York) government is entering the fray, a promising development that is indeed welcome. So, at present, when one is purchasing any of these products, he/she is running the risk of not only suffering from a toxic ingredient, but also receiving little or nothing (which may be a blessing in disguise).

A major difference between a drug and a dietary supplement is that dietary supplements may not claim to "diagnose, cure, mitigate, treat, or prevent specific illnesses." Consequently, dietary supplement manufacturers can make only general "structure/function" claims, which are often vaguely worded assertions of health benefits such as "support the body's natural defenses", "promote heart health," "better circulation," "increased energy," "better joint health and mobility," etc. They regularly provide a disclaimer that their product "has not been evaluated by the Federal Drug Administration (FDA)." Their wording is regularly evasive, for claims to treat specific diseases cause products to be considered drugs. Firms making such assertions legally must follow FDA's premarket new drug approval process to show the products are both safe and effective—an onerous and expensive task.

Conclusion:

I would strongly warn everyone to avoid all these products, for if you don't, you may be literally taking your life in your own hands.

If, however, you are determined to consume any of these products and wish to ascertain whether you are getting what the label actually claims, a few independent non-profit organizations test for purity from voluntarily provided samples. One organization is the United States Pharmacopeia, which allows an official and distinctive black and yellow "USP Verified" seal to be affixed after satisfactory results are obtained. A second such group is NSF International, which provides a blue and white NSF seal that means that a product has been independently vetted to ensure that it is not adulterated and that it contains the ingredients listed on its label. Lastly, there are at least two independent laboratories that routinely test a range of dietary supplements and then publish reports with their findings. They are ConsumerLab.com and LabDoor, which test many products and maintain an archive of reports on their websites, but they come with a fee.

If, however, you wish to determine whether a given supplement may be risky, go to the search box at www.fda.gov to see whether it has been subject to warnings, alerts, or voluntary recalls. If you suspect you're having a bad reaction to a supplement, tell your doctor. You can also report your problem to the FDA at 800-332-1088 or www.fda.gov/medwatch. What is far better, however, is to avoid these so-called supplements altogether in favor of eating a decent diet.

CHAPTER 57

Alkaline Water: Another Scam Designed To Take Your Money

If you believe the marketing hype, alkaline water can increase your energy, boost your metabolism, hydrate you better than regular water, prevent digestive problems, neutralize acid in your bloodstream, help your body absorb nutrients more effectively, promote weight loss, prevent bone loss, and even slow aging. But is there any reality in all this?

What is Alkaline Liquid?

You may already know that the term pH actually stands for the potential for hydrogen. That's what the P and the H mean. In chemistry, it is a measure of the acidity or alkalinity of an aqueous solution. Solutions with a pH less than 7 are said to be acidic, and solutions with a pH greater than 7 are basic, or alkaline. Pure water has a pH very close to 7, which is neutral. Human blood is slightly alkaline, with a nearly constant Ph value of 7.4. So if a liquid is 7.5, you can say it's alkaline. If it's 8.5 it's alkaline, and so on.

Water Can Be "Alkalized"

Alkaline water is commonly produced by an "ionizer." In alkaline ionizers, an electrolysis process separates the water into two parts, or sides: One side is alkaline – this stream of water is used for drinking, and the pH is over 7. The other side is acidic, i.e., possesses a pH below 7, but is not dealt with here.

The Body Has Ways Of Providing Balance

Our bodies are wonderful machines. If there is an imbalance, we have ways to correct it. Unless you have certain conditions such as kidney or respiratory disease, your body maintains a healthy pH balance on its own. For example, once an alkaline liquid hits your stomach, the acidic gastric juices will neutralize it, providing an example of natural balancing. Skewing your body's pH balance too far in either direction—too acidic or too alkaline — can cause problems. Your body wants something close to neutral, and it has numerous ways of achieving it. Because adequate hydration is crucial for health, we all should consume liberal amounts of plain water and avoid dehydration. But there is actually no scientific justification for imbibing alkalinized water.

Alkaline Ionizers Don't Make Safe Drinking Water

Most people don't realize that the actual **source of water** is the critical factor, and an alkaline ionizer doesn't remove contaminants. Thus one needs to be aware of what is present or absent in the water's source. Alkaline ionizers are not water purifiers and have no sophisticated technology and no real filtration ability, which sellers often hype. Thus alkaline ionizers are an expensive proposition (they can cost up to $7,000) for absolutely no real physical benefit.

Conclusion:

Alkaline ionizers do not contribute to acid-alkaline balance in your body (or alkalizing your blood stream). The body needs no help with this job.

Alkaline ionizers are not good filters. Your drinking water could still contain contaminants that are unsafe to drink.

Alkaline ionizers are unnecessarily expensive. Why spend thousands on this process when you can have more success with pure, clean water?

No scientific studies have demonstrated any advantage to modifying water in this way.

ᴄᴈᴑCHAPTER 58ᴄᴐᴑ

Human Growth Hormone to Prevent Aging: Yet Another Snake Oil

In a segment of one of his shows, the celebrated TV host, Dr. Oz, began by asking his audience, "How many of you want to start feeling 20 years younger right now?" Then, after hearing the predictable chorus of yes's, he went on to discuss what he called "a new frontier: stimulating your body's production of growth hormones naturally with amino acids." And then Dr. Oz told his adoring audience, "I have been searching for this from the day we started the show. I've been looking for ways of increasing HGH naturally because I don't like getting the injections." As is his customary style, he then started a new frenzy of those wishing to seek out such a product, in this case called "SeroVital."

But what does this all mean? Human growth hormone, or HGH, is a natural substance secreted by a small gland (pituitary) in the brain. It promotes growth during childhood and adolescence. Growth hormone acts on the liver and other tissues to stimulate the production of insulin-like growth factor I (IGF-I), which is responsible for its growth-promoting effects. Blood levels of circulating IGF-I tend to decrease as people age or become obese. Many marketers would like you to believe that boosting HGH blood levels can reduce body fat; build muscle; improve sex life, sleep quality, vision and memory; restore hair growth and color; strengthen the immune system; normalize blood sugar; increase energy; and "turn back your body's biological clock." Unfortunately all this not only lacks experimental support but is patently false, as will be summarized below. This has also been aptly described in greater detail by Stephen Barrett, MD, the editor of the popular website, Quackwatch, which I strongly recommend.

The drive to popularize growth hormone began about 20 years ago with publication of the book "Life Extension: A Practical Scientific Approach," by Pearson and Shaw. These authors claimed that large amounts of vitamins, minerals, amino acids, and other substances would cause people to add muscle, burn fat, and live much longer. Although their advice had no scientific basis, these authors made hundreds of talk-show appearances that boosted sales of the products they recommended.

Soon after the book's publication, many amino acids were claimed to cause overnight weight loss by increasing the release of growth hormone. So called "growth-hormone releasers" were also marketed to bodybuilders with claims that they would help build muscle. Such claims are unfounded because amino acids taken by mouth do not produce such effects. These formulations are based mainly on misinterpreted studies of intravenous arginine, which can increase HGH blood levels for an hour or so. The FTC and the New York City Department of Consumer Affairs attacked some companies making "growth-hormone release" claims, but these actions had very little effect on the overall marketplace.

In 1990, *The New England Journal of Medicine* published a study that attracted mainstream media attention. The study involved 12 men, aged 61 to 81, who were apparently healthy but had IGF-I levels below those found in normal young men. The 12 men were given growth hormone injections three times a week for six months and were compared with 9 men who received no treatment. The treatment resulted in a decrease in fatty tissue and increases in body muscle mass and spine density An accompanying editorial warned that some of the subjects had experienced side effects and that the long-range effects of administering HGH to healthy adults were unknown. It also warned that the hormone injections were expensive and that the study had not examined whether the men who received the hormone had actually improved their muscle strength, mobility, or quality of life.

In March 2003, in response to growing controversy, the *New England Journal of Medicine* took the unprecedented step of denouncing misuse of the above mentioned 1990 article. The full text of the article was placed online so readers could see for themselves what it actually said; and editorials pointed out that subsequent reports provided no reason to be optimistic. As noted by Editor-in-Chief Jeffrey M. Drazen, M.D.:

"Although the findings of the study were biologically interesting, the duration of treatment was so short that side effects were unlikely to have emerged, and it was clear that the results were not sufficient to serve as a basis for treatment recommendations"

Indeed, Mary Lee Vance of the University of Virginia said in an accompanying editorial *"Because there are so many unanswered questions about the use of growth hormone in the elderly and in adults with growth hormone deficiency, its general use now or in the immediate future is not justified."*

Despite these reservations, the initial study of 1990 inspired many offbeat care givers to market themselves as "anti-aging specialists." offering expensive tests that supposedly determine the patient's "biological age." They promised to lower this "age," with expensive hormone shots and dietary supplements. To this date, nobody has provided any evidence that it is more than just another myth.

All this hype also helped stimulate formation of the American Association for Anti- Aging Medicine and the unrecognized medical specialty of "anti-aging medicine." The group, founded in 1993, claims that it has 11,500 members, of whom 80% are medical or osteopathic physicians. Many exhibitors at its conferences have made unsubstantiated claims for HGH-related products.

Also springing up are thousands of Web sites and spam e-mailers that are hawking the actual hormone for oral use (which can't work because HGH itself cannot pass the intestinal barrier to reach the bloodstream).

But what we do know thus far is simply that HGH is useful for treating growth hormone deficiency in children and adults and has a few other proven but limited (FDA-approved) uses. The American Association of Clinical Endocrinologists has warned that the clinical use of growth hormone for any patient—with or without ordinary obesity—is not recommended and could possibly lead to unknown dangers.

Robert N. Butler, M.D., a noted gerontologist who founded a legitimate organization, the International Longevity Center-USA, has warned that, "So-called anti-aging medicine is largely a sham. We simply do not have the equivalent of a blood pressure cuff for testing aging." He further states:

Although growth hormone levels decline with age, it has not been proven that trying to maintain the levels that exist in young persons is beneficial. It is conceivable that age-related hormonal changes may serve as useful markers of physiological aging. However, this has not been demonstrated experimentally for either humans or animals. Although hormone-replacement trials have yielded some positive results (at least in the short term), it is clear that negative side effects can also occur in the form of increased risk for cancer, cardiovascular disease, and behavior changes.

It might even turn out that lower growth-hormone levels are an indicator of health. Research findings indicate that mice that overproduce growth hormones live only a short time, suggesting that growth-hormone deficiency itself does not cause accelerated aging, but that the opposite may be true.

In short, physicians have no scientifically based measures of aging, and lacking this indicator, there is no way to fight against something that can't be identified.

So how can ingesting "HGH stimulators" produce any benefits? From the foregoing, the answer is apparent—they cannot! Although growth hormone levels decline with age, there is no proof that trying to maintain the levels that exist in young persons is beneficial. Considering the high cost, significant side effects, and lack of proven effectiveness, HGH injections appear to be a very poor investment. So called "growth-hormone releasers," "oral growth hormone," and "homeopathic HGH" products are thus clearly fakes.

Into this category we place the product noted above touted by Dr. Oz, manufactured by SanMedica International under the trade name SeroVital. Even if this product could stimulate HGH production by the body, which is doubtful, any long-term benefits from such stimulation are totally unproven, and are likely to remain so for a long time in the future.

Sure, it's tempting to try every product on the market that promises a more youthful look and feel, but sometimes good, old fashioned diet and exercise can have the same effect as a "miracle pill."

CHAPTER 59

Scams Presented By the "Legitimate" Drug Companies

Are you tired of being bombarded by the drug ads on TV urging you to "ask your doctor about prescribing a particular drug" for your problem? More accurately stated, they actually mean "pressure your doctor into prescribing our very expensive drug in order to fatten our income, and possibly even help your condition."

But are such disingenuous tactics working? Unfortunately, aggressive marketing is persuading many people to overpay for medication. According to IMS Health, a pharmaceutical intelligence company which tracks drug sales and marketing, drug makers spent $4.3 billion to reach consumers and $6.6 billion on promotions aimed at both patients and physicians. These tactics seem to be succeeding. *Consumer Reports* states that, in a recent poll, 20% of respondents said they asked for a drug they'd learned about from advertising, and 59% of those said their doctor agreed to write a prescription for that product. So I must admit that even many members of my own profession share some of the blame for such questionable practices.

Let's cite some of the more blatant examples of pharmaceutical misrepresentation:

Example 1: AndroGel (testosterone). A middle aged man proclaims his relief when a doctor says that his moodiness and low energy were caused by "Low T," and therefore, he required treatment with testosterone. Unfortunately, although testosterone levels in the blood fall normally with age, the symptoms noted above are far more likely to be caused by depression, anxiety, obesity, and other problems. Thus before embarking on testosterone treatment, careful—usually repeated—testing of the blood is required, and this is better supplemented by the advice of a specialist in glandular disorders (endocrinologist). Although the dangers of such treatment have been previously suspected, we now have more confirmation that testosterone therapy taken for "low T" raises the risk of mortality, heart attacks and strokes, according to recent study.[87] Because of this potential risk, the FDA has issued a warning (2015) that requires labeling changes for all prescription testosterone products.

Example 2: Humira (adalimumab). A woman is embarrassed by her psoriasis (skin condition) when visiting a new hair salon. After asking her physician about Humira, she is then shown enjoying less stress and better skin when visiting that same beauty salon.

The down side: This drug is a potent agent useful for severe arthritic diseases and inflammatory conditions of the bowel. It is very expensive and must be given by injection. Possible severe (even life-threatening) side effects may occur because it interferes with the body's immune system. One must undertake such a treatment under much caution, and not generally for gaining a more acceptable skin appearance.

Example 3: Crestor (rosuvastatin). A doctor describes the dangers of LDL (bad cholesterol) in contributing to plaque buildup in arteries. He says that in a clinical trial, Crestor helped more high-risk patients get their LDL below 100 in comparison with other similar ("statin") drugs. The real story:

While Crestor is a very strong drug, it doesn't really matter which of the several statin drugs are used to lower the blood levels as long as the goal levels are reached. Thus a cheaper alternative to Crestor may suffice quite well to get to the desired goal and, therefore, confer just as much protection against bad cardiovascular outcomes. Crestor is better reserved for those instances in which the other drugs (such as generic lovastatin) cannot attain the targeted goal.

Example 4: Cymbalta (duloxetine). Men and women with arthritis or low-back pain are told that Cymbalta, a non-narcotic pain reliever, can help. Cymbalta is also recommended for several other conditions such as depression, anxiety, and other causes of pain.

The real truth: Cymbalta flunks in all categories. Regarding relief of back pain and various forms of arthritis, it is less effective than the commonly used non-steroidal anti-inflammatory drugs (NSAIDS) such as ibuprofen (Advil), which are far cheaper. Moreover, Cymbalta is no more effective for depression than other, less expensive drugs for this purpose. Bottom line: There is hardly any justification for the use of this drug against anything.

Example 5: Celebrex (celecoxib): A man is playing in the snow with his family. Having taken Celebrex for his arthritis, he is now quite active. This drug is a member of the group of "non-steroidal anti-inflammatory drugs" (NSAID). Celebrex differs from the older varieties such as ibuprofen (Advil) by possessing a lower propensity to cause gastrointestinal upset or ulceration. But what's the catch? Celebrex's pain relief is no greater than that of the older generics. If one is able to tolerate these latter drugs without gastrointestinal problems, that's the best choice. Stomach irritation from the cheap generics can be avoided by simply taking them with food or antacids. Moreover, Celebrex can increase the chances for cardiovascular problems such as heart attacks. Although some studies have implicated the older generics in cardiovascular problems, their incidence appears to be lower, if present at all. So, in general, opt for the generics if they agree with your gastrointestinal system and you haven't had past problems with ulcers or intestinal bleeding.

Conclusion:

From the information provided above: Whenever encountering any pharmaceutical ad, you might be better served by ignoring it altogether. If you actually do ask your doctor about the advertised product, inquire first if there is a cheaper generic alternative that is likely to be just as effective.

CHAPTER 60

Beware of the Media Health "Authorities"
Who is an "Authority?"

We all encounter pronouncements by "authorities" (often self-proclaimed scientists) who claim something about almost anything. Upon exploring the issue further, we discover that we have no idea who these people are and whether they possess any qualifications to back up their claims. A series of letters following a name does not automatically confer one's right to claim anything. For instance, an MD or PhD after a name suggests that some basic qualifications are present, but almost everyone is subject to biases, errors, and hidden motives—often driven by conflicts of interest. With regard to "scientists," Brian Dunning, popular author and skeptical pod-caster, aptly stated, "The fact that calling someone a scientist doesn't mean that he's smart, that he's right, that he thinks scientifically, or that he's anything more than a waste of space. All this means is that the label of 'scientist' is pretty damned worthless by itself." But how can an average individual avoid being seduced by such slick salesmen?

First, we should always be skeptical of any assertions that seem questionable or improbable, especially when financial gain or products is involved. When possible, try to determine the origin of any assertions, which may quickly expose the validity, weakness, or absence of underlying facts. If you are unable or unqualified to verify this information, seek the opinions of recognized authorities qualified in the same field of endeavor. Actually, Google is a good starting point, but avoid those entries that have something to sell and try to find impartial sources such as Wikipedia and academic institutions.

Unfortunately, some "authorities," with or without scientific credentials, appear to gain credibility through their entry into the media, especially television. Their mere presence seems to confer an air of validity to whatever they are saying (or selling). So let's take a look at a recent study of televised medical talk shows that appeared in a respected medical journal entitled *Televised medical talk shows—what they recommend and the evidence to support their recommendations: A prospective observational study*[88]. The investigators evaluated 80 episodes from *The Dr Oz Show* and *The Doctors* from early 2013, selecting recommendations made from each program.

These researchers concluded the following:

1.   For recommendations in The Dr Oz Show, evidence supported 46%, contradicted 15%, and was inconclusive for 39%.

2.   For recommendations in The Doctors, evidence supported 63%, contradicted 14%, and was inconclusive for 24%.

3.   "Believable" or "somewhat believable" evidence supported 33% of the recommendations on The Dr Oz Show and 53% on The Doctors.

But this is only a small sample of so much mischief reverberating in our media. Both Dr. Mehmet Oz and Dr. Travis Stork and his co-hosts (*The Doctors*) are licensed physicians, but despite their credentials, seem to be willing to dispense unproven, false, or misleading information. Many other so-called "authorities" lack these credentials and, as you might anticipate, dole out even more misinformation to an unsuspecting—and often uncritical—public.

Dr. Oz merits special recognition. One of his transgressions—but not the most outrageous—follows a charge brought by the U.S. Federal Trade Commission (FTC) that he is involved in a scam to deceive consumers through fake news sites and bogus weight loss claims: He recently touted the use of green coffee bean dietary supplement as a potent weight loss treatment that supposedly burns fat. The FTC alleged that weeks after Oz's promotion, several individuals, who control various companies—NPB Advertising, Inc. and others—began marketing through sites that featured excerpts from Oz's show and testimonials from "consumers" who were paid for their participation. They also set up sites that featured mastheads of fictitious news organizations such as Women's Health Journal and Healthy Living Reviewed, as well as logos they appropriated from actual news organizations, like CNN and MSNBC. The FTC charged the defendants with falsely claiming that users of their product could lose 20 pounds in four weeks, 16% of body fat in 12 weeks, and 30 pounds and four-to-six inches of belly fat in 3 to 5 months. "Not only did these defendants trick consumers with their phony weight loss claims, they also compounded the deception by advertising on pretended news sites, making it impossible for people to know whether they were seeing news or an ad," said Jessica Rich, Director of the FTC's Bureau of Consumer Protection.

But such revelations are really nothing new: Oz was recognized by the James Randi Educational Foundation (JREF) that promotes critical thinking through grants for outstanding educators, scholarships to inspire skeptical students, and annual conferences showcasing the best of skeptical thought. Every April Fools Day, this organization "honors the five worst offenders who are intentionally or unintentionally pulling the wool over the public's eyes, providing awards to the most deserving charlatans, swindlers, psychics, pseudo-scientists, and faith healers—and to their credulous enablers, too". The awards are named for both the mythical flying horse Pegasus of Greek mythology and the highly improbable flying pig (Pigasus) of popular cliché. In 2009 and 2011, the *Pigasus Award* went to Dr. Mehmet Oz, and I quote *"who has done such a disservice to his TV viewers by promoting quack medical practices that he is now the first person to win a Pigasus award for two years. Dr. Oz, through his syndicated TV show, has promoted faith healing, energy medicine, and other quack theories that have no scientific basis. Oz has appeared on ABC News to give legitimacy to the claims of Brazilian faith healer 'John of God,' who uses old carnival tricks to take money from the seriously ill. He's hosted Ayurvedic guru Yogi Cameron on his show to promote nonsense 'tongue examination' as a way of diagnosing health problems. In March 2011, Dr. Oz endorsed 'psychic' huckster and past Pigasus winner John Edward, who pretends to talk to dead people. Oz even suggested that bereaved families should visit psychic mediums to receive (faked) messages from their dead relatives as a form of grief counseling. "*

Finally, in 2015, ten prominent academic physicians from prestigious medical institutions called Columbia University to remove Oz from his academic position there because of his advancement of sometimes dangerous advice and unfounded "quack" treatments. In fighting back, Oz defended his position by falling back on his First Amendment rights and stating "My job, I feel, on the show is to be a cheerleader for the audience when they don't think they have hope." Instead, however, he seems to be promoting false hope. Departing from the dictates of principled medical ethics, Oz appears to have lost his way, and may not be such a great "wizard" after all, not unlike the movie character that was exposed for what he was after the curtain was removed from all his misleading master controls!

But such disingenuous information extends beyond TV to news reports, books and more, presented by "authorities" with or without credentials, and they may be even more misleading than those TV programs mentioned above. "Doctor diet books" seem to be special offenders: Examples of these are the so-called Atkins diet, promulgated by Robert Atkins, MD. Having no special background in dietetics, Atkins derived his recommendations after reading a single report entitled "A New Concept in the Treatment of Obesity", that was published in a 1963 issue of the *Journal of the American Medical Association*. Atkins never published any of his own data in peer-reviewed journals, and the soundness of his dietary claims has been repeatedly questioned by many qualified authorities. More recently, I encountered a book by Wm Davis, MD, a physician from Milwaukee, entitled "Wheat Belly," which claims that our consumption of wheat gluten can be blamed not only for overweight but also such unrelated conditions as depression, eating disorders, migraine headaches, diabetes, high cholesterol, skin rashes, joint pain, and many others. Scientific basis for any of these claims— zero! Gluten from wheat can be blamed for an intestinal disorder called "celiac disease," found in only a tiny percentage (about 1%-2%) of our population. I have summarized the actual scientific information on this condition in chapter 39.

I could go on and on, but I believe the message is clear.

Bottom Line

Consumers should be skeptical about any recommendations provided on television medical talk shows or other media outlets, as details are limited. In the case of the TV shows noted above, only a third to one half of recommendations are based on believable evidence. In the case of medical talk shows, an interesting question is whether we should expect them to provide anything more than just entertainment. If the shows are perceived as providing medical advice, viewers need to realize that the recommendations may not be supported by solid evidence or presented with enough balance to adequately make decisions with regard to health. These issues are often challenging and require far more than non-specific recommendations from media health professionals. Thus, again, buyers beware!

CHAPTER 61

"Detoxifying" The Body of Unwanted Substances: Another Blatant Scam!

The idea of "detoxifying" or "purifying" the body of "harmful" substances has been around for centuries and returns periodically to haunt the modern world. The idea behind such "cleansing" schemes is to rid the body of some unknown substance(s)— usually vaguely specified, sometimes promising to rid the system of "toxins" absorbed from the environment and the less-than-healthy foods we eat.

The basic concept of "detoxifying" is blatantly flawed, for our natural processes, especially liver and kidney function, cleanse our bodies far better than any extrinsic activities or substances could possibly achieve. Some detox ideas center also on the intestines, but by attempting to flush out the "bad stuff" from our intestines, they are also threatening to flush out the good bacteria that keep the intestines healthy, which is becoming a hot topic these days (chapter 44).

The various plans can last anywhere from three days to about a month or more. In the process of flushing "poisons" from your body, they promise to eliminate pounds of excess fat, clear your complexion and bolster your immune system, while leaving you feeling more energized. While believers claim they feel more energetic, studies on starvation show the longer you fast, the more lethargic and less focused you become.

Very often these ideas are popularized by "experts" in alternative medicine, i.e., quacks. There are no hard numbers on how many people have tried the latest fashionable plans, much less stuck with them, but dozens of new do-it-yourself cleansing or fasting books are glutting bookstore shelves. Each of the programs has its own take on how to cleanse the body— one calls for spices and fruit juices, another for only vegetable purees—but most of them boil down to extremely low-calorie, primarily liquid diets.

Some plans restrict all solid foods and instruct dieters to survive on only low-calorie beverages for days at a time. The Joshi holistic diet involves an elaborate list of so-called "acid-forming foods" to avoid for three weeks, including healthy vegetables and grains.

Those plans that include lengthy or repeated fasts, or near-fasts, pose, in themselves, significant risks. Nutritional deficiencies are serious drawbacks. Some plans that restrict solid foods often call for laxatives, resulting in frequent liquid bowel movements. If a fast lasts for several weeks, it may lead to muscle breakdown and a shortage of many needed nutrients, depriving the body of the vitamins and minerals obtained from food. Thus, in contrast to the claimed benefits, it can actually weaken the body's ability to fight infections and inflammation. Also, because most of these diets contain very little protein, it can be difficult to rebuild lost muscle tissue

Because many crash diets can upset blood sugar, potassium and sodium levels in the body, they should be strenuously avoided by anyone with diabetes, heart or kidney disease, or by women who are pregnant or nursing. Children, teens, older adults or people with certain digestive conditions should also steer clear.

Unfortunately, many of these plans include various herbal products that are not carefully monitored by the FDA. These various components have recently been associated with an increasing rate of toxic effects, most notably liver injury (chapter 56).

One of the latest detoxifying vogues is that of "Detox Tea," which purports to rid the body of unspecified "toxins." One promoter of these teas states that, "In the modern world, we're exposed to many pollutants like caffeine, smoke and food toxins. These pollutants accumulate in the body and cause our overall health to decline. Drinking detox tea helps to remove these toxins from the body. It does this by supporting the internal cleansing process by adjusting the fire and air energies." How vague can this be? The same source also clarifies that "detox tea is made from with a combination of herbs and spices, which has been used for centuries in India. The actual ingredients are cinnamon, liquorice, ginger, dandelion, fennel, anise, juniper berries, burdock root, coriander, cardamom, parsley, sage, cloves, turmeric root, and black pepper. Also, detox tea is caffeine free and contains a laxative." I suppose that all it lacks is a partridge in a pear tree.

The same "detox tea" company then goes on to issue a mild disclaimer: "Claims that drinking detox tea is good for the liver, lungs and kidneys are difficult to verify. These claims have not been verified by the Food and Drug Administration, and because of this, no one should rely on detox tea to treat or prevent disease. Also, despite the fact that detox tea is advertised as a health food, drinking it will not help you lose weight." This is clearly a defensive statement, designed to keep the "feds" off of their tails. Similar statements are issued on virtually all bogus products that have not been supported by acceptable scientific proof.

Conclusion:

I would simply advise the public to steer clear of this entire concept of "detoxification." The idea is simply presented to take your money while lacking scientific proof of benefit. But even more distressing, as noted above, there is often no good way to find out whether any of these products poses a danger to health.

ᑲ᠊CHAPTER 62ᑫᓕ

Standard Medical Care or Chiropractic Treatment?

An interesting quotation recently appeared in Consumer Health Digest, well-known for its exposure of medical and health scams. Consumer Health Digest is a free weekly e-mail newsletter edited by Stephen Barrett, M.D, who also edits another well-respected site, Quackwatch. It summarizes scientific reports; legislative developments; enforcement actions; news reports, web site evaluations; recommended and non-recommended books; and other information relevant to consumer protection and consumer decision-making.

The quotation to which I refer was obtained from software engineer Dan Kegel who discovered a 61-page manual from the Chiropractic Business Institute that appears to have circulated in the 1950s.

This chiropractic manual unearthed by this publication states as follows:

In addition to technique, there are four other factors of vital importance. You must also be a master salesman, an astute psychologist, a brilliant individualist, and an able business man.

All doctors are naturally familiar with Diagnosis, but its interpretation means only the diagnosing of disease. Yet there is a second diagnosis of equal and vital importance. It deals primarily with analyzing a patient from a business standpoint, to determine his worth to the doctor.

Many of the sales pitches are geared toward:

1. *Persuading patients to continue to have weekly care long after their symptoms have resolved.*

2. *Undermining trust in medical doctors.*

3. *Promoting chiropractic for preventing as well as treating the gamut of health problems.*

These themes are still common in currently available chiropractic practice-building courses. Moreover, although the present code of ethics for such practitioners omits this verbiage in favor of high-sounding generalizations, many chiropractors conduct themselves in a way consistent with the principles noted above.

But what is the underlying philosophy behind the entire field of chiropractic treatment? As Benedetti and MacPhail explain in their book entitled "Spin Doctors: The Chiropractic Industry Under Examination," the chiropractic field lacks any unifying principles, the majority clinging slavishly to an outdated concept of a mythical spinal condition "subluxation," to which they attribute all kinds of maladies extending from back and muscular pains to include internal organs in both adults and children. Chiropractors often espouse unproven methods that include a breathtaking array of whacky devices and methods such as "Activator, Neurocalcometer, Applied Kinesiology, Reflexology, Interro and Vegatest machines," extending to other unproven techniques such as cranial sacral therapy, homeopathy herbalism, acupuncture, vitamin and supplement therapy, and much more—too numerous to list here. Benedetti and MacPhail go on to state rightly that, "Nothing specific to chiropractic has been shown to be of any health benefit, a statement that has been true for over 100 years. Spinal manipulative therapy that may be effective in the treatment of a small range of short-lived low-back pain can be done by other therapists who are better educated, just as skilled, and not encumbered by decades of anti-scientific dogma and irrational beliefs." With regard to low back pain persisting for over 12 weeks, a recent analysis[89] of studies comparing spinal manipulation with prescribed exercise revealed no conclusive evidence favoring one over the other. Only three randomized controlled trials met the inclusion criteria of the review: One favored manipulation, one favored exercise, and the third study judged them equal. Surprisingly, this review was presented in a chiropractic journal.

Finally Benedetti and MacPhail state that, chiropractors, feeling themselves as representatives of a major justified alternative route of "medical" care, often suggest that there is a "battle between chiropractic and medicine. That's untrue. The real battle is between science and science fiction." They add further that; "What really matters is that chiropractic has betrayed its patients' trust. The chiropractic profession is always playing what is best for the patient against what is best for chiropractic. Most often, the patient loses."

The doctrine quoted above appears perversely inimical to the principles espoused by the vast majority of my colleagues licensed to practice conventional medicine across the entire U.S., and these contrasts are worth noting.

As a member of the mainstream medical community, I and others have always sworn to the principles embodied in the so-called *Hippocratic Oath* that dates back to ancient Greece. Since then, the oath has been modified numerous times.

I quote below the major portions of modern version of this oath, which was last modified in the 1960s:

I swear to fulfill, to the best of my ability and judgment, this covenant:

I will respect the hard-won scientific gains of those physicians in whose steps I walk, and gladly share such knowledge as is mine with those who are to follow.

I will apply, for the benefit of the sick, all measures which are required, avoiding those twin traps of overtreatment and therapeutic nihilism.

I will remember that there is art to medicine as well as science, and that warmth, sympathy, and understanding may outweigh the surgeon's knife or the chemist's drug.

I will not be ashamed to say "I know not," nor will I fail to call in my colleagues when the skills of another are needed for a patient's recovery.

I will respect the privacy of my patients, for their problems are not disclosed to me that the world may know. Most especially must I tread with care in matters of life and death. If it is given me to save a life, all thanks. But it may also be within my power to take a life; this awesome responsibility must be faced with great humbleness and awareness of my own frailty. Above all, I must not play God.

I will remember that I do not treat a fever chart, a cancerous growth, but a sick human being, whose illness may affect the person's family and economic stability. My responsibility includes these related problems, if I am to care adequately for the sick.

I will prevent disease whenever I can, for prevention is preferable to cure.

I will remember that I remain a member of society, with special obligations to all my fellow human beings, those sound of mind and body as well as the infirm.

If I do not violate this oath, may I enjoy life and art, respected while I live and remembered with affection thereafter. May I always act so as to preserve the finest traditions of my calling and may I long experience the joy of healing those who seek my help.

Today this oath is taken by virtually all my fellow practitioners. While there is currently no legal obligation for medical students to swear an oath upon graduating, 98% of American medical students swear to this exact form, or to a comparable oath. In the United States, osteopathic physicians are now included in the groups committed to providing science-based care, and the majority of osteopathic medical schools use either a similar Oath or this Hippocratic Oath. While it is not legally binding, the oath provides principles of conduct that codify ethical/professional standards. Although exceptions do occur in this imperfect world, failure to adhere to any of these principles places a heavy burden on one's own conscience, and opens one up to censure by his/her peers. On the other hand, chiropractors are not included in this form of scientific-based care-giving, nor do they subscribe to a comparable oath.

I leave it to the reader's discretion regarding where to place his/her faith: one who has sworn to follow this latter oath, or to someone committed to alternative principles.

Conclusion:

Issues of human health and its care are divided primarily into two parallel universes:

1.   Science-based medicine, espoused by the vast majority of licensed physicians and care-givers throughout the entire world.

2.   Alternative medicine, which comprises a large conglomeration of unproven remedies, along with a variety of practitioners bearing numerous titles, which sometimes seem to convey an apparent scientific air of legitimacy. But, as time elapses, the two universes are drifting further apart, leaving vast rifts between the receding tectonic plates. Below we examine some issues about both these universes.

Evidence Based Medicine

This form of medicine is based upon sound scientific principles, involving careful observations of both individuals and groups. Most contemporary scientific research, however, involves studying groups of individuals, then usually employing statistical analyses of varying complexity to determine which relationships are meaningful and which are chance occurrences. This requires plain knowledge of statistical principles and their proper application. But not all problems fit neatly into well-defined pigeonholes; which means that I—as a practitioner—in order to reach the best conclusions, must exercise my best judgment based upon principles learned through background, education, and experience.

Research studies, after completion, are generally submitted to peer-reviewed journals in order to gain general acceptance. This means that, to be published, they must be reviewed and accepted by "peers," i.e., qualified scientists that possess qualifications that enable them to judge the merits of any given project. Since this system is not infallible, results often require confirmation by other similar studies performed in other institutions or places. Thus the correct final conclusions are usually arrived at by a confirmatory process. This renders the entire system—although cumbersome—usually self-correcting.

During the past half century, we have witnessed tremendous advances in medical science, involving the understanding of basic bodily functions, diagnostic procedures and technology, and treatments of all types. Virtually all these remarkable advances are attributable to the principles of scientific evidence, employed extensively primarily in this latter time period.

But the evidence-based system has various disadvantages[90]:

Because of delays in publication and confirmation, it tends to be relatively slow-moving.

One form of distortion is produced by "publication bias," i.e. preferential publication of "positive" results. We know that reports of test outcomes are more likely to be accepted by scientific journals when they demonstrate "positive" outcomes—the apparent success of any given treatment or procedure. Conversely, negative findings are seldom considered as an initial offering by standard journals; they are simply not as appealing, or "groundbreaking," as are those that are positive. The editors themselves also have some stake in these acceptances, for publishing "striking" results can confer an aura of prestige to their journal. Critical analyses[91,92] have shown that trials with positive findings, i.e., showing statistically significant outcomes perceived to be important with positive effects of treatment—had nearly four times the odds of being published compared to findings that were perceived as unimportant or showed a negative direction of the treatment effect. These studies also disclosed that trials with positive findings also were published more quickly than trials with negative findings. Adding to this problem, media reporters may further amplify the findings through a process of "spin," defined as specific reporting strategies that emphasize the beneficial effect of an experimental treatment. In one systematic study[93], "spin" was detected in about half of a large number of press and media releases. In detailed analysis, the main factor associated with the "spin" in these releases seemed to emanate primarily from positive conclusions in the abstracts in the research articles themselves, but undoubtedly the reporters also played a role in this overemphasis, since this would likely enhance their own aggrandizement or that of their publication.

Interference by pharmaceutical companies or equipment makers tends to create bias in reporting by suppressing results that are less favorable to their products. This deficiency has been at least partially addressed by the U.S. Government, which has recently required entry of all large randomized studies of drugs and devices into a common database (ClinicalTrials.gov). But this attempt to eliminate exclusion of studies was limited because, of a number of large trials that were prospectively registered in ClinicalTrials.gov and completed before January 2009, only 50% had published results.[94] This leaves us with a large hiatus in knowledge about many large clinical trials—that portion with the greatest potential impact on clinical care.

Errors in the performance of research occasionally creep into the picture, and this sometimes leads to subsequent published retractions, a tendency that has been increasing in recent years[95].

But despite these and a few other drawbacks, medical science has shown an admirable track record during this scientific era and has kept pace with the rapidly developing fields of computer science, engineering, geology, etc. Because of the many factors noted above, however, the average person should be critical when initial media reports indicate major "advances" or "breakthroughs." Very often subsequent study tempers or invalidates these findings, sowing the seeds of considerable later disappointment.

Alternative Medicine

Alternative medicine may be defined as any healing practice that does not fall within the realm of conventional medicine. It is based on historical or cultural traditions, rather than on scientific evidence, and it has features resembling faith or spiritual healing. This definition includes a broad array of therapeutic interventions unstudied by conventional contemporary methods, and so it operates apart from evidence based medicine.

Angell and Kassirer[96] best sum up the feeling of the scientific community toward alternative medicine:

It is time for the scientific community to stop giving alternative medicine a free ride. There cannot be two kinds of medicine—conventional and alternative. There is only medicine that has been adequately tested and medicine that has not, medicine that works and medicine that may or may not work. Once a treatment has been tested rigorously, it no longer matters whether it was considered alternative at the outset. If it is found to be reasonably safe and effective, it will be accepted. But assertions, speculation, and testimonials do not substitute for evidence. Alternative treatments should be subjected to scientific testing no less rigorous than that required for conventional treatments.

These authors state further that alternative medicine also distinguishes itself by an ideology that largely ignores biologic mechanisms, often disparages modern science, and relies on what are purported to be ancient practices and natural remedies, which are seen as being simultaneously more potent and less toxic than conventional medicine. Thus herbs or mixtures of them are considered superior to active compounds isolated in the laboratory. Notwithstanding these statements, unorthodox healing methods continue to be fervently and widely promoted.

Singh and Ernst, in their book entitled *Trick or Treatment: The undeniable facts about alternative medicine*[97], have aptly summarized this situation with the statement, "Conventional medicine and alternative medicine both have the same ambition, namely to cure the sick, and yet one is tightly regulated and the other operates in the medical equivalent of the Wild West. This means that patients who venture towards alternative medicine are at risk of being exploited, losing their money and damaging their health."

The fields of alternative medicine include, among others, chiropractic treatment, herbalism, traditional Chinese medicine, ayurvedic medicine, meditation, yoga, biofeedback, hypnosis, homeopathy, acupuncture, nutritional-based therapies, holistic medicine, energy medicine, and reflexology.

Some alternative medicine methods are added to conventional approaches. Then it is defined as *complementary/alternative medicine* (CAM). According to Steven Novella, editor of the website Science-Based Medicine, "this expression is a political/ideological entity, not a scientific one." Nevertheless, this approach, although unjustified in my opinion, has been included in the services offered by many U.S. hospitals.

Although alternative methods are largely employed by non-conventional and unlicensed practitioners, occasional licensed physicians step across these boundaries and promote alternative methods, as described in chapter 60. In my opinion and that of most of my colleagues, this is a risky, if not dangerous, step that can produce more harm than good.

Unfortunately, even our U.S. and state governments are accomplices in contributing, however unwittingly, to the perpetuation and growth of the "alternative industry" through the creation of the National Center for Complementary and Integrative Health (NCCIH), the licensing and supporting of those individuals, methods and institutions as described in chapter 53. The impotence of the overstressed and underfunded FDA, is also a contributor by virtue of its inability to provide adequate surveillance of the various dietary "supplements" that are ubiquitous in our environment.

But why do such large segments of the public seem to accept uncritically these unsubstantiated methods and claims? Although not amenable to any single answers, I have described two major factors[98] that seem to explain much of this acceptance: Perhaps the most important factor is the so-called *placebo effect*[99], that is, any improvement in subjective discomfort or illness not explained by the effect of the treatment given. This effect originates in the brain and is not well understood, but can exhibit improvements that are actually felt physically. Given the proper circumstances, such as positive expectations or the application of active personal contact or procedures, this effect can be quite powerful indeed. The second factor accounting for apparent "treatment" success is that most illness and pain subside spontaneously. Thus any intervention—no matter how farcical—that precedes improvement will often receive full credit for the favorable outcome. When these apparent "cures" are related anecdotally to others, this throws more fuel on the fire, consequently spreading misconceptions far and wide.

Although I am a member of the conventional medical community, I believe that our relative silence on this subject also has contributed to the ongoing acceptance of these alternative, oftentimes fraudulent, methods. We need to be active participants in the process of "whistle blowing" in the effort to bring our public and governmental agencies into 21st century thought processes. Although we are often cynically accused of protecting our own financial turf by condemning these non-scientific methods, this is clearly false! I agree with most of my colleagues that our main concerns are subservient to the public interest, and, in the process, helping those who waste large resources on useless—sometimes dangerous—techniques and treatments.

It is my hope that this book will, at least in some small way, contribute to the process of enlightenment.

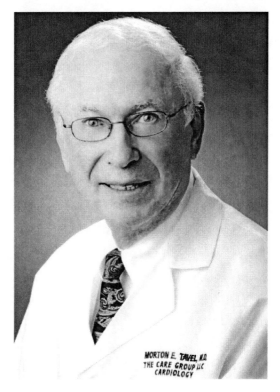

About The Author

ow retired, Dr. Tavel MD, FACP, FACC, was a physician specialist in internal medicine and cardiovascular diseases. In addition to managing patients for many years, he held a teaching position (Clinical Professor) at Indiana University School of Medicine. He was consulting cardiologist for the Care Group, Inc., a division of St. Vincent Hospital in Indianapolis and was the director of the cardiac rehabilitation program. His civic activities include, among others, having been past president of the local and Indiana state divisions of the American Heart Association.

He has presented numerous speeches and lectures before national audiences. His medical research includes over 120 publications, editorials, and book reviews that have appeared in peer-reviewed national medical journals. Dr. Tavel authored a book on cardiology (Clinical Phonocardiography) that persisted through four editions over a period of approximately 20 years, and has been a contributor to several other multi-authored textbooks. He has served on the editorial boards of several national medical journals. Recent books are noted below.

Recent Books

Snake Oil is Alive and Well: The Clash between Myths and Reality. Reflections of a Physician. Brighton Publishing, LLC, Mesa, Ariz., 2012

Hell in the Heavens: The Saga of a WW2 Bomber Pilot, by Tavel, ME and Tavel, DE. Brighton Publishing, LLC, Mesa, Ariz. 2013.

Health Tips, Myths and Tricks: A Physician's Advice. Brighton Publishing, LLC, Mesa, Ariz. 2015.

References

[1] "BMI Classification". *Global Database on Body Mass Index.* World Health Organization. 2006. Retrieved in 2012 by Wikipedia,

[2] Johnston BC et al. Comparison of Weight Loss among named diet programs in overweight and obese Adults. A meta-analysis *JAMA.* 2014;312(9):923-933.

[3] Galsziou P, et al, Pre-meal water consumption for weight loss Aust Fam Physician. 2013 Jul;42(7):478.

[4] Cahill LE. et al. Prospective study of breakfast eating and incident coronary heart disease in a cohort of male US health professionals. *Circulation.* 2013;128:337-343.

[5] Betts JA, et al. The causal role of breakfast in energy balance and health: a randomized controlled trial in lean adults. Am J Clin Nutr. 2014 doi: 10.3945/ajcn.114.083402

[6] Ibid

[7] Honors A. Trends in Fatty Acid Intake of Adults MN Metropolitan Area, 1980–1982 Through 2007–2009 *J Am Heart Assoc. 2014; 3* J Am Heart Assoc. *2014; 3: e001023 doi: 10.1161/JAHA.114.001023*

[8] O'Keefe JH, Bhatti SK, Patil HR, et al. Effects of habitual coffee consumption on cardiometabolic disease, cardiovascular health, and all-cause mortality. J Am Coll Cardiol 2013;62:1043-51.

[9] Gang L and Xiaohong H. Effects of tea intake on blood pressure: a meta-analysis of 21 randomized controlled trials Journal of the American College of Cardiology.Volume 64, Issue 16, Supplement, 21 October 2014, Page C112

[10] Pang J, et al Green tea consumption and the risk of the related factors of cardiovascular diseases and ischemic related diseases: A meta-analysis. International Journal Cardiology. 1/12/2015. DOI: http://dx.doi.org/10.1016/j.ijcard.2014.12.176. Published online: January 3, 2015

[11] Nurk E, Refsum H, Drevon CA, et al. Intake of flavonoid-rich wine, tea, and chocolate by elderly men and women is associated with better cognitive test performance. J Nutr 2009;139:120-127.

[12] Messerli FH. Chocolate consumption, cognitive function, and Nobel laureates. N Engl J Med 367;16:1562-1564.

[13] Adriana Buitrago-Lopez, et al. Chocolate consumption and cardiometabolic disorders: systematic review and meta-analysis. BMJ 2011; 343:d4488

[14] Wang C, Fang C, Chen N, et al. Cranberry-containing products for prevention of urinary tract infections in susceptible populations. *Arch Intern Med.* 2012;172(13):988-996

[15] Cassidy A, et al "High anthocyanin intake is associated with a reduced risk of myocardial infarction in young and middle-aged women" *Circulation* 2013;112.122408.

[16] Devore E.E., et al. *Dietary intakes of berries and flavonoids in relation to cognitive decline* Annals of Neurology.2012;72:135-143.

[17] Poole DC et al. Skeletal muscle capillary function: contemporary observations and novel hypotheses. Exp. Physiol.2013;98:1645-1658.

[18] Ghosh SM et al Enhanced vasodilator activity of nitrite in hypertension: critical role for erythrocytic xanthine

oxidoreductase and translational potential. Hypertension. 2013 May;61(5):1091-102.

[19] Queen Mary University of London News, 01/21/2015

[20] Ros E. and Hu FB. Consumption of plant seeds and cardiovascular health. Epidemiological and clinical trial evidence. Circulation 2013;128:553-565.

[21] Bao Y. et al. Association of nut consumption with total and cause-specific mortality. N. England J. Med. 2013;369:2001.

[22] Nutrition Action Health letter, July/August 2013

[23] Jacobson M.F. and McCarter R. Changes in sodium levels in processed and restaurant foods, 2005 to 2011. JAMA Internal Medicine. 173;20134:1285-91

[24] Campbell's Soup, ConAgra Foods, Domino's Pizza, General Mills, Hormel Foods Corp., McDonald's, Smithfield Hams, Sodexo, Inc., Subway, and Walmart

[25] An Pan, et al. Red Meat Consumption and Mortality Results From 2 Prospective Cohort Studies. *Arch Intern Med.* 2012;172(7).2011: 555-563

[26] Holmes et al. Association between alcohol and cardiovascular disease: Mendelian randomization analysis based on individual participant data: BMJ 2014;349:g4164

[27] Tome-Carneiro J., Gonzalvez, M, Larrosa M, et al. One-year consumption of a grape nutraceutical containing resveratrol improves the inflammatory and fibrinolytic status of patients in primary prevention of cardiovascular disease. Am J Cardiol 2012;110:356-363.

[28] Gulliford MC, et al. Continued high rates of antibiotic prescribing to adults with respiratory tract infection: survey of

568 UK general practices *BMJ Open 2014;4:e006245 doi:10.1136/bmjopen-2014-006245.*

[29] Hemila H and Chalder E. The effectiveness of high dose zinc acetate lozenges on various common cold symptoms: a meta analysis. *BMC Family Practice* 2015, 16:24

[30] Gardner C. et al. Nonnutritive Sweeteners: Current Use and Health Perspectives A Scientific Statement from the American Heart Association and the American Diabetes Association Circulation. 2012;126:509-519.

[31] Swithers SE. Artificial sweeteners produce the counterintuitive effect of inducing metabolic derangements. Trends

[32] Fowler SPG, Williams K, and Hazuda HP. Diet Soda Intake Is Associated with Long-Term Increases in Waist Circumference in a Biethnic Cohort of Older Adults: The San Antonio Longitudinal Study of Aging. *Journal of the American Geriatrics Society*; Published Online: March 17, 2015 (DOI: 10.1111/jgs.13376)

[33] The health consequences of smoking: 50 years of progress: a report of the Surgeon General. 2014.

(http://www.surgeongeneral.gov/library/reprorts/50years-of-progress/#fullreport)

[34] Carter BD et al.. Smoking and mortality—Beyond established causes. N Engl J Med 2015;372:631-640.

[35] Glantz SA and Gibbs E. Changes in ambulance calls after implementation of a smoke-free law and its extension to casinos. *Circulation*. 2013;128:811-813.

[36] Hart JE, et al. Changes in Traffic Exposure and the Risk of Incident Myocardial Infarction and All-Cause Mortality Epidemiology.2013; 24(5):734–742.

[37] Puett, RC. Particulate Matter Air Pollution Exposure, Distance to Road, and Incident Lung Cancer in the Nurses' Health Study Cohort. Environ Health Perspect. 2014; 122(9): 926–932

[38] Bullen C. et al. Electronic cigarettes for smoking cessation: a randomized controlled trial.. Lancet 2013; 382;1629–1637.

[39] Cobb NK and Abrams DB. The FDA, E-Cigarettes, and the Demise of Combusted Tobacco N Engl J Med 2014; 371:1469-1471.

[40] Hughes MC, et. al. Sunscreen and Prevention of Skin Aging: A randomized trial. Annals of Internal Medicine. 2013;158:781-790.

[41] Roussel NA, Nijs J, Meeus M. et al. Central Sensitization and Altered Central Pain Processing in Chronic Low Back Pain Clin J Pain 2013;29:625–638

[42] Koes BW, van Tulder MW, and Thomas S. Diagnosis and treatment of low back pain. BMJ. 2006 Jun 17; 332(7555): 1430–1434

[43] Linton SJ, Hallden K. Can we screen for problematic back pain? A screening questionnaire for predicting outcome in acute and subacute back pain. Clin J Pain 1998;14: 209-15

[44] Tavel ME, Snake Oil is Alive and Well: The Clash between Myths and Reality. Reflections of a Physician. Brighton Publishing, Mesa, Arizona, 2012

[45] Ibrahim T, Tleyjeh IM, and Gabbar O. Surgical versus non-surgical treatment of chronic low back pain: a meta-analysis of randomized trials...Int Orthop 2008; 32:107–113.

[46] Fitzgerald JD, et al. Association of Objectively Measured Physical Activity with Cardiovascular Risk in Mobility-

limited Older Adults. *Journal of the American Heart Association*, 2015; 10.1161

[47]http://www.cancer.gov/cancertopics/factsheet/prevention/physicalactivity

[48] Kampert JB, et al. Physical activity, physical fitness, and all-cause and cancer mortality: a prospective study of men and women. Ann Epidemiology. 1996;6::452-7.

[49] DeFina LF, et al. The Association Between Midlife Cardiorespiratory Fitness Levels and Later-Life Dementia: A Cohort Study *Ann Intern Med* 2013;158(3):162-168

[50] Erickson KI, Raji CA, Lopez OL, et al. Physical activity predicts gray matter volume in late adulthood: the Cardiovascular Health Study. Neurology. 2010;75:1415-1422

[51] Khan, N.A, et al. Impact of the FITKids physical activity intervention on adiposity in prepubertal Children. Pediatrics:2014:10.1542

[52] Kelly M. Naugle, Roger B. Fillingim, and Joseph L. Riley, III A meta-analytic review of the hypoalgesic effects of exercise. J Pain. 2012; 13(12): 1139–1150.

[53] Jones MD, et al. Aerobic training increases pain tolerance in healthy individuals.Med Sci Sports Exerc. 2014 Aug;46(8):1640-7

[54] Wheatley LM and Togias A. Allergic Rhinitis. N. Engl J Med. 2015;372(5):456-463.

[55] Oliver JE, Wood T. Medical conspiracy theories and health behaviors in the United States. JAMA Internal Medicine, 2014;174(5):817-818

[56] Wakefield AJ. MMR vaccination and autism. Lancet. 1999; 354:949–950

[57] Nyhan B. et al. Effective messages in vaccine promotion: A randomized trial. Pediatrics, 2014;.133(4):e835-842

[58] Smith-Spangler CS, Brandeau MS, Hunter GE, et al. Are Organic Foods Safer or Healthier Than Conventional Alternatives? A Systematic Review. Ann Intern Med. 2012;157(5):348-66.

[59] Sengupta P. Potential Health Impacts of Hard WaterInt J Prev Med. Aug 2013; 4(8): 866–875.

[60] Cunrui Huang, The Hygienic Efficacy of Different Hand-Drying Methods: A Review of the Evidence. Mayo Clinic Proceedings. 2012;87:791–798

[61] Best E. Potential for aerosolization of Clostridium difficile after flushing toilets: the role of toilet lids in reducing environmental contamination risk. J Hosp Infect. 2012;80(1):1-5.

[62] Barker J The potential spread of infection caused by aerosol contamination of surfaces after flushing a domestic toilet. J Appl Microbiol. 2005;99(2):339-47.

[63] Purcell K. The effect of rate of weight loss on long-term weight management: a randomised controlled trial. Lancet. Diabetes and Endocrinology 2014;2:954-962

[64] Hampton T. Infection and Air Travel. *JAMA.* 2005;293(20):2463.

[65] Mangili A. and Gendeau M. Transmission of infectious diseases during commercial air travel. Lancet. 2005:365, 989–996

[66] Iacono, W.G. "Forensic 'lie detection': Procedures without scientific basis," *Journal of Forensic Psychology Practice,* 2001;(1):75-86

[67] Reid JE, Inbau FE. 1977. Truth and deception: The polygraph ("lie detector") technique. Williams & Wilkins, Baltimore

[68] Saxe L, Dougherty D, Crosse T. 1983. Scientific validity of polygraph testing: a research review and evaluation. *Conference: OTA-TM.* U.S. Congress Office of Technology Assessment

[69] Lykken DT. Why (some) Americans believe in the lie detector while others believe in the guilty knowledge test. *Integrative Physiological and Behavioral Science.* 1991;26: 214-222.

[70] Horvath F. 1977. The effect of selected variables on interpretation of polygraph records. *Journal of Applied Psychology.* 62: 127-136.

[71] Brett AS, Phillips M, Beary JF. 1986. Predictive power of the polygraph: Can the "lie detector" really detect liars? *The Lancet.* 1: 544-547.

[72] Kleinmuntz B, Szucko J. 1984. A field study of the fallibility of polygraphic lie detection. *Nature.* 308: 449-450

[73] Lykken D. 1984. Polygraph Interrogation. *Nature.* 307: 681-684.

[74] Lykken DT. 1981. A tremor in the blood: Uses and abuses of the lie detector. McGraw-Hill, New York.

[75] Lykken DT. 1991. Why (some) Americans believe in the lie detector while others believe in the guilty knowledge test. *Integrative Physiological and Behavioral Science.* 26: 214-222.

[76] Tavel ME, Snake Oil is Alive and Well: The Clash between Myths and Reality. Reflections of a Physician. Brighton Publishing Mesa, Ariz., 2012, p. 51

[77] Iacono, WG. Forensic Lie Detection: Procedures Without Scientific Basis, *Journal of Forensic Psychology Practice,* 2001;(1):75-86

[78] Gergley JC. Acute effect of passive static stretching on lower-body strength in moderately trained men J Strength Cond Res. 2013:973-7.

[79] Krogsbøll LT. General health checks in adults for reducing morbidity and mortality from disease Published Online: 17 OCT 2012 DOI: 10.1002/14651858.CD009009.pub2

[80] Bloomfield HE. Screening Pelvic Examinations in Asymptomatic, Average-Risk Adult Women: An Evidence Report for a Clinical Practice Guideline From the American College of Physicians. Ann Intern Med. 2014;161:46-53

[81] Mielczarek E. and Engler BD. Measuring mythology: Startling concepts in NCCAM grants. Skeptical Inquirer 36(1):35-43,. 2012

[82] Tavel ME. The Placebo Effect: The Good, The Bad, and The Ugly. The American Journal of Medicine. 2014; 127(6):484–488.

[83] Mielczarek E. and Engler BD. Measuring mythology: Startling concepts in NCCAM grants. Skeptical Inquirer 36(1):35-43,. 2012

[84] Sampson, W.I. Why the National Center for Complementary and Alternative Medicine (NCCAM) Should Be Defunded, 2002. http://www.quackwatch.org/01QuackeryRelatedTopics/nccam.htl

[85] Jiratchariyakul W and MahadyGB Overview of botanical status in EU, USA, and Thailand Evidence Based Complement Alternat Med. 2013; 480128. Published online Oct 21, 2013. doi: 10.1155/2013/480128

[86] Harel Z et al. The Frequency and Characteristics of Dietary Supplement Recalls in the United States. *JAMA Intern Med.*, 2013 DOI:

[87] Finkle WD et al. Increased Risk of Non-Fatal Myocardial Infarction Following Testosterone Therapy Prescription in Men. PLoS One. 2014; 9(1): e85805. Published online 2014

[88] Korownyk C et al. Televised medical talk shows—what they recommend and the evidence to support their recommendations: a prospective observational study BMJ 2014; 349 doi: http://dx.doi.org/10.1136/bmj.g7346

[89] Merepeza A. Effects of spinal manipulation versus therapeutic exercise on adults with chronic low back pain: a literature review. J Can Chiropr Assoc 2014; 58(4);456-465.

[90] Tavel ME. Bias in Reporting of Medical Research: How Dangerous is It? Skeptical Inquirer. 2015;39(3):34-38

[91] Dwan K, et al. Systematic Review of the Empirical Evidence of Study Publication Bias and Outcome Reporting Bias — An Updated Review Published online Jul 5, 2013. 10.1371/journal.pone.0066844. PMCID: PMC3702538

[92] Jones CW, Handler L, Crowell KE, et al. BMJ. 2013; 347: f6104. Non-publication of large randomized clinical trials: cross sectional analysis.Published online Oct 29, 2013

[93] Yavchitz A, et al. Misrepresentation of Randomized Controlled Trials in Press Releases and News Coverage: A Cohort Study. PLoS Med 9(9): e1001308. doi:10.1371/journal.pmed.1001308

[94] Riveros C, et al. Timing and Completeness of Trial Results Posted at ClinicalTrials.gov and Published in Journals PLoS Med. Dec 2013; 10(12): e1001566. Published online Dec 3, 2013

[95] Tavel ME. *Snake Oil is Alive and Well*. Brighton Publishing, Mesa, Ariz. 2012, p. 199.

[96] Angell M, Kassirer JP. Alternative medicine—the risks of untested and unregulated remedies The New England Journal of Medicine 1998; 339:839–41

[97] Singh S. and Ernst E. *Trick or Treatment: The undeniable facts about alternative medicine.* W.W. Norton Co. New York and London, 2008. p. 281.

[98] Tavel ME. Snake Oil is Alive and Well: The Clash between Myths and Reality. Reflections of a Physician. Brighton Publishing, Mesa, Arizona, 2012.

[99] Tavel ME. The Placebo Effect: The Good, The Bad, and The Ugly. The American Journal of Medicine. 2014; 127(6):484–488

CPSIA information can be obtained
at www.ICGtesting.com
Printed in the USA
FSOW01n2338200217
30959FS

9 781621 833406